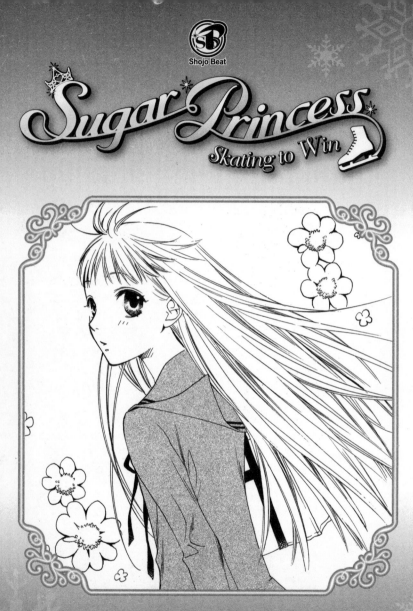

Story & Art by
Hisaya Nakajo

Vol. **1**

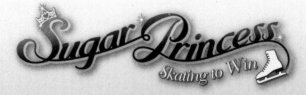

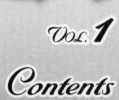

Contents

Men's Singles

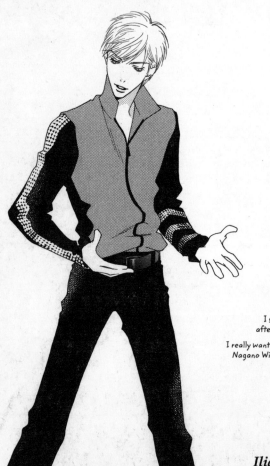

I love Kulik!
I still love him even
after he turned pro... ↘

I really wanted to go see him at the
Nagano Winter Olympics, but...

Ilia KULIK

Sugar Princess
Skating to Win

Chapter 1

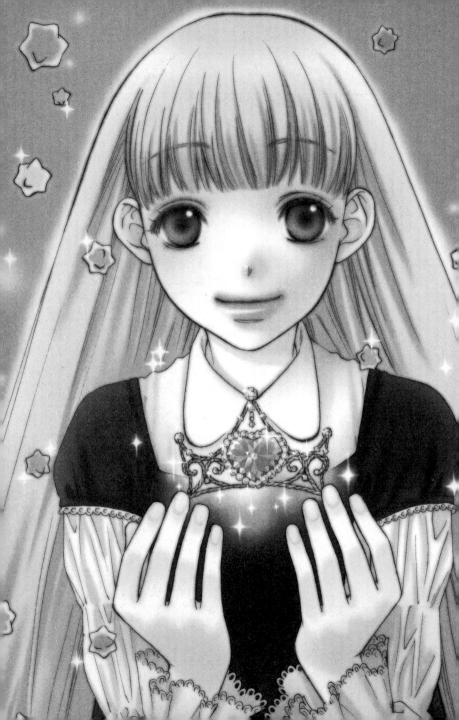

Women's Singles

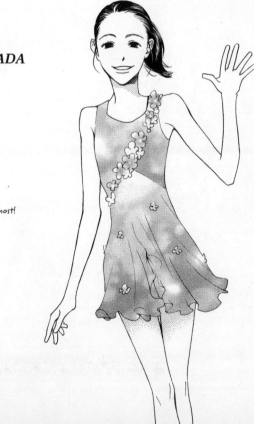

Mao ASADA

I'm rooting for Mao the most!
Go, Mao!

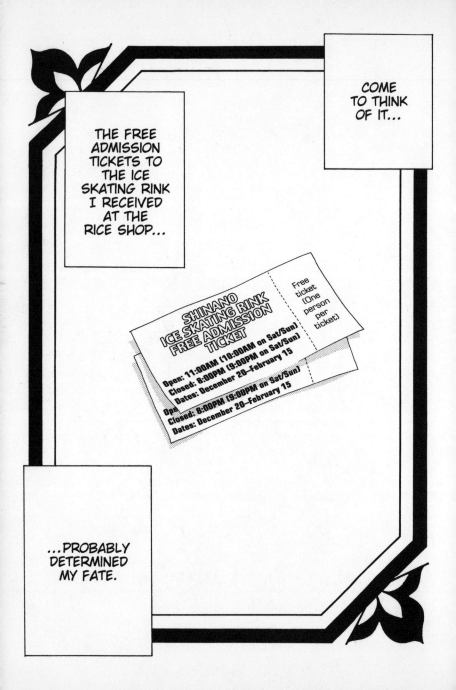

COME TO THINK OF IT...

THE FREE ADMISSION TICKETS TO THE ICE SKATING RINK I RECEIVED AT THE RICE SHOP...

SHINANO
ICE SKATING RINK
FREE ADMISSION
TICKET

Free ticket (One person per ticket)

Open: 11:00AM (10:00AM on Sat/Sun)
Closed: 8:00PM (9:00PM on Sat/Sun)
Dates: December 20–February 15

Ope
Closed: 8:00PM (9:00PM on Sat/Sun)
Dates: December 20–February 15

...PROBABLY DETERMINED MY FATE.

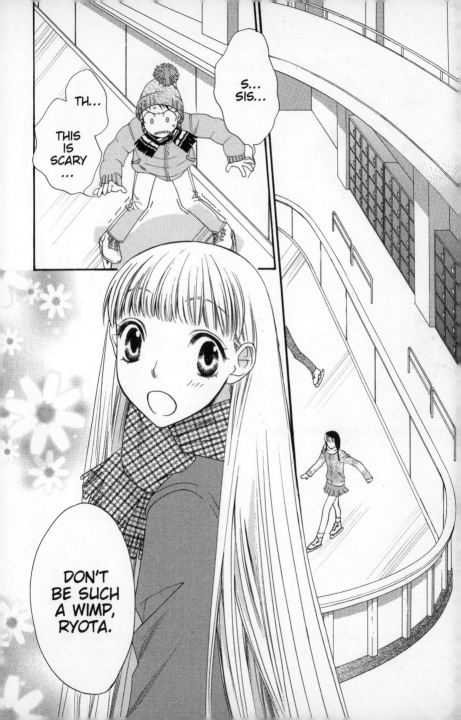

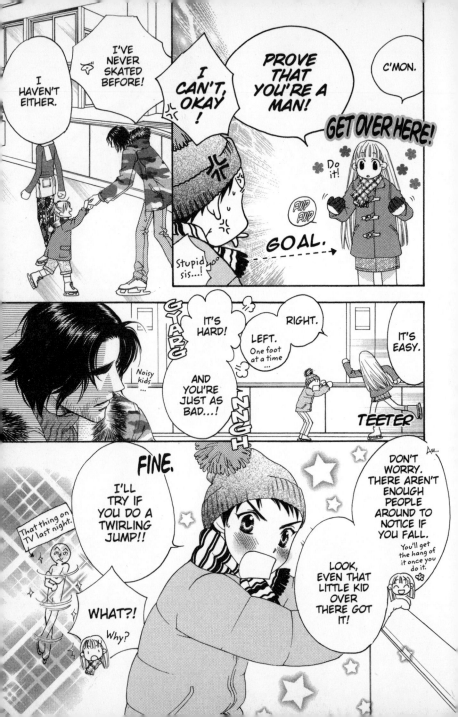

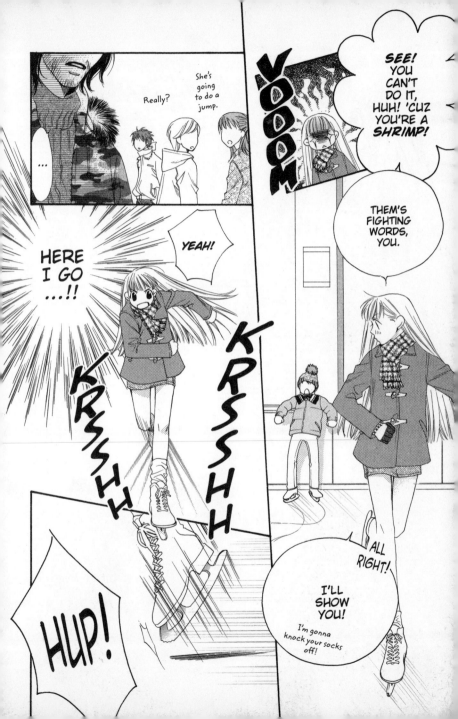

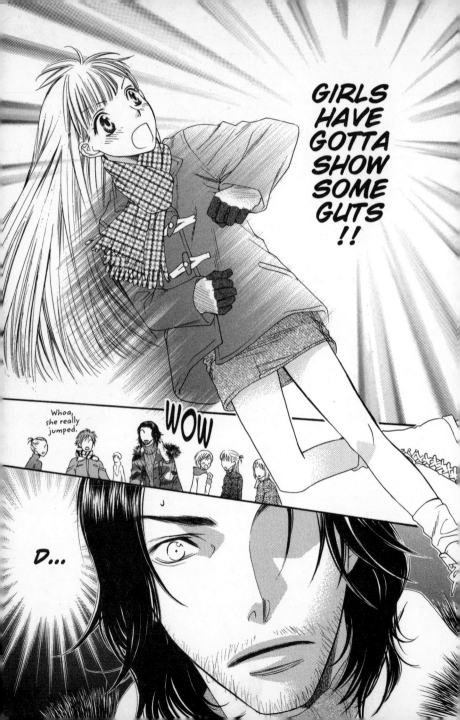

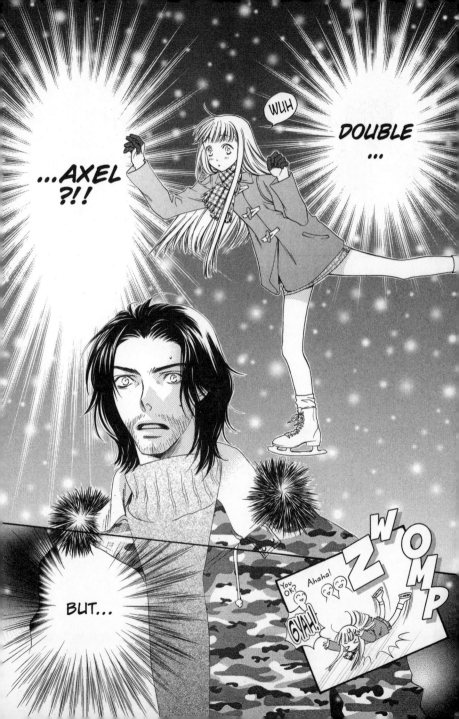

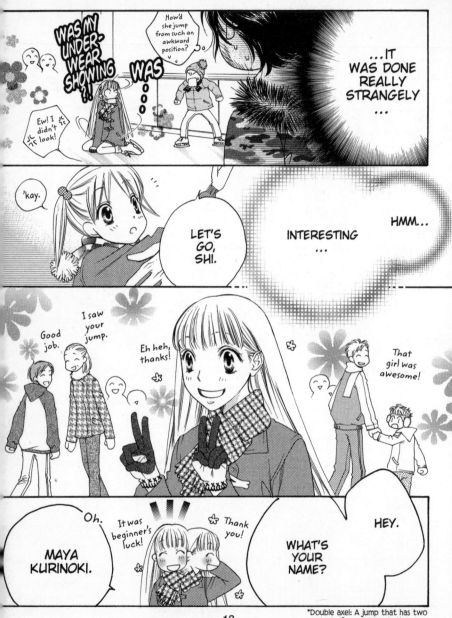

WAS MY UNDERWEAR SHOWING?!

WAS...

How'd she jump from such an awkward position?

Ew! I didn't look!

...IT WAS DONE REALLY STRANGELY...

'kay.

LET'S GO, SHI.

INTERESTING...

HMM...

Good job.

I saw your jump.

Eh heh, thanks!

That girl was awesome!

Oh.

It was beginner's luck!

Thank you!

HEY.

MAYA KURINOKI.

WHAT'S YOUR NAME?

13

*Double axel: A jump that has two and a half revolutions in the air.

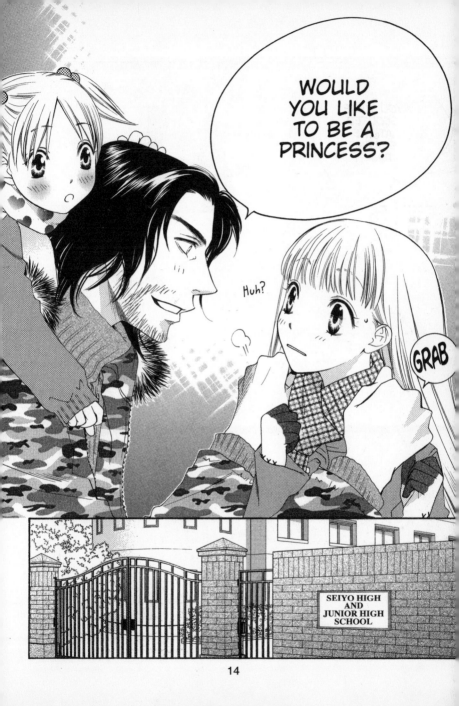

14

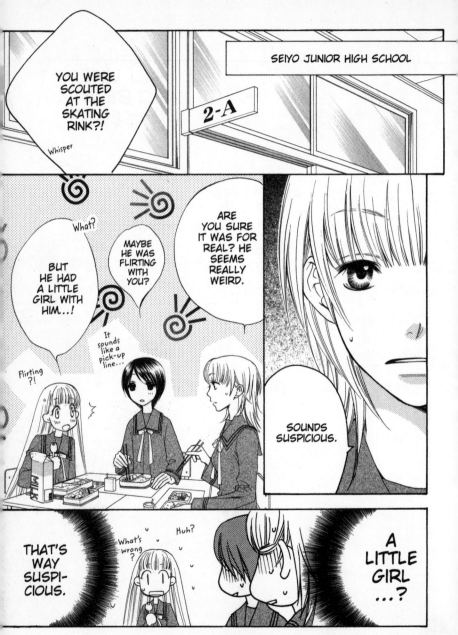

SEIYO JUNIOR HIGH SCHOOL

2-A

YOU WERE SCOUTED AT THE SKATING RINK?!

Whisper

What?

MAYBE HE WAS FLIRTING WITH YOU?

ARE YOU SURE IT WAS FOR REAL? HE SEEMS REALLY WEIRD.

BUT HE HAD A LITTLE GIRL WITH HIM..!

It sounds like a pick-up line...

Flirting ?!

SOUNDS SUSPICIOUS.

MILK

THAT'S WAY SUSPI-CIOUS.

What's wrong?

Huh?

A LITTLE GIRL ...?

15

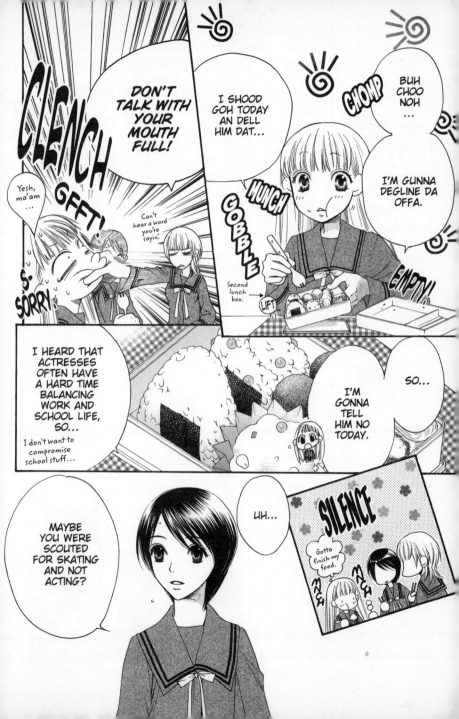

CLENCH

GFFT!

DON'T TALK WITH YOUR MOUTH FULL!

Yesh, ma'am...

S. SORRY

Can't hear a word you're sayin'!

I SHOOD GOH TODAY AN DELL HIM DAT...

CHOMP

BUH CHOO NOH...

MUNCH

GOBBLE

LIFT

Second lunch box.

I'M GUNNA DEGLINE DA OFFA.

EMPTY!

I HEARD THAT ACTRESSES OFTEN HAVE A HARD TIME BALANCING WORK AND SCHOOL LIFE, SO...

I don't want to compromise school stuff...

I'M GONNA TELL HIM NO TODAY.

SO...

MAYBE YOU WERE SCOUTED FOR SKATING AND NOT ACTING?

UH...

SILENCE

Gotta finish my food.

MNCH

MNCH

THAT'S PROBABLY IT.

YOU'RE RIGHT, NANAKO!...

I ONLY THOUGHT OF ACTING SCOUTS...

How embarrassing...

GOSH... OF COURSE!

AND WHY ME...?

MAYA.

WHERE DO YOU NEED TO GO TO DECLINE THE OFFER?

A SPORTS SCOUT, HUH? THEN WHICH SKATING EVENT WAS I SCOUTED FOR?

OH!

HE GAVE ME A BUSINESS CARD. HE WANTED ME TO DISCUSS IT WITH MY PARENTS.

LET'S SEE THE CARD.

I'M A LITTLE CURIOUS...

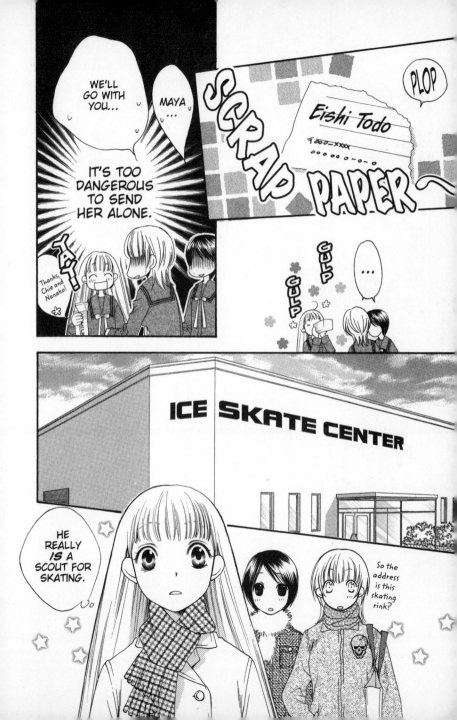

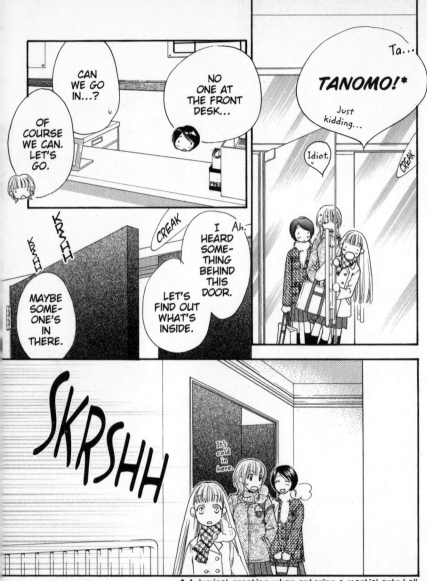

* A typical greeting when entering a martial arts hall

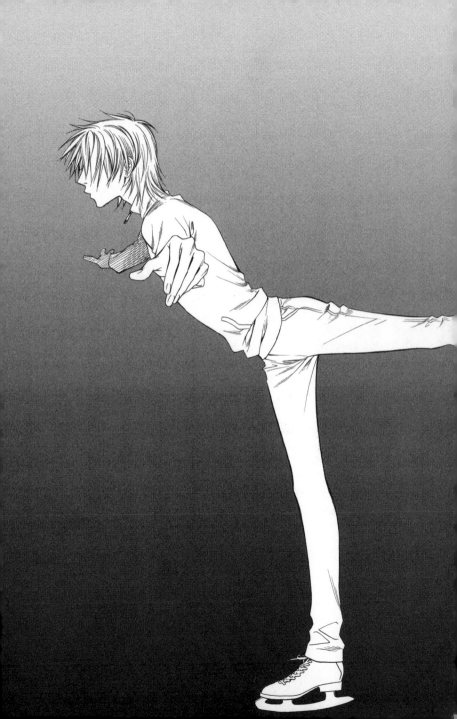

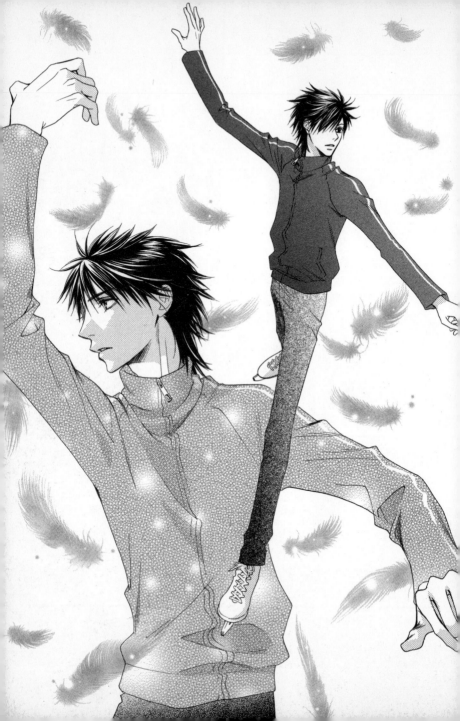

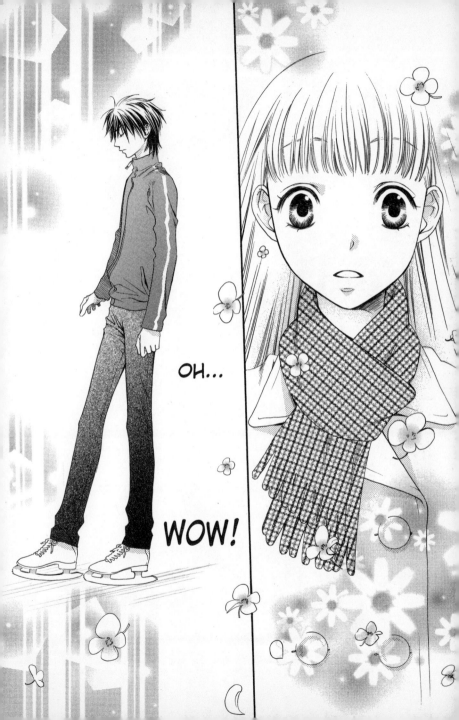

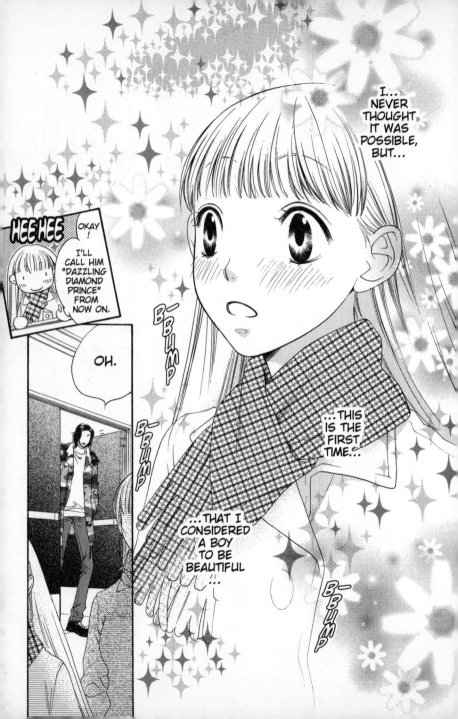

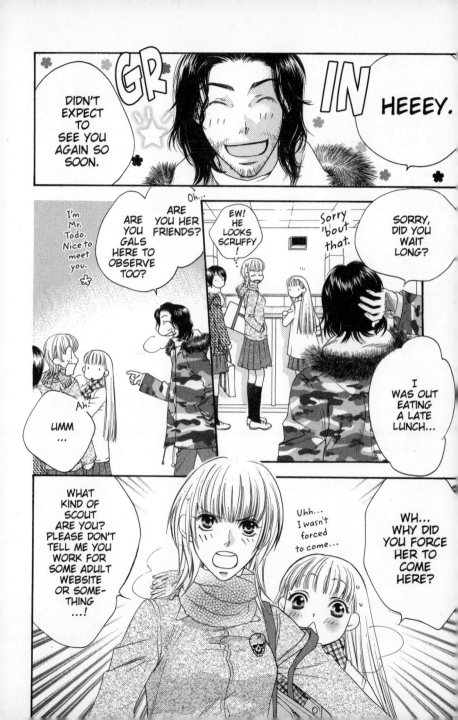

DIDN'T EXPECT TO SEE YOU AGAIN SO SOON.

GR IN

HEEEY.

I'm Mr. Todo. Nice to meet you. ❀

ARE YOU GALS HERE TO OBSERVE TOO?

ARE YOU HER FRIENDS?

Oh...

EW! HE LOOKS SCRUFFY!

...

Sorry 'bout that.

SORRY, DID YOU WAIT LONG?

I WAS OUT EATING A LATE LUNCH...

Ah...

UMM...

WHAT KIND OF SCOUT ARE YOU? PLEASE DON'T TELL ME YOU WORK FOR SOME ADULT WEBSITE OR SOME-THING ...!

Uhh... I wasn't forced to come...

WH... WHY DID YOU FORCE HER TO COME HERE?

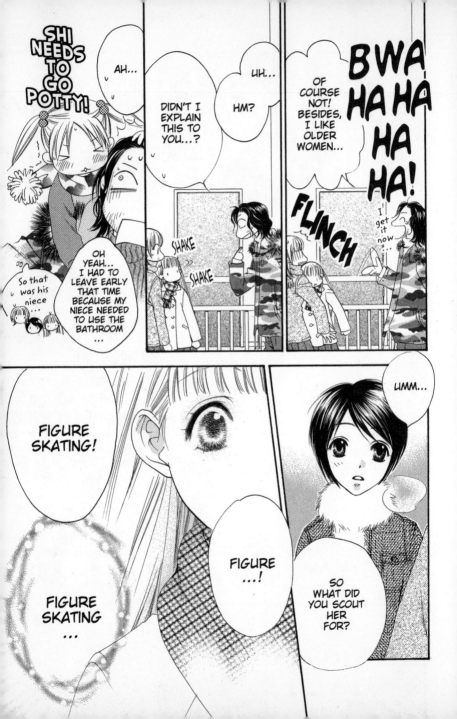

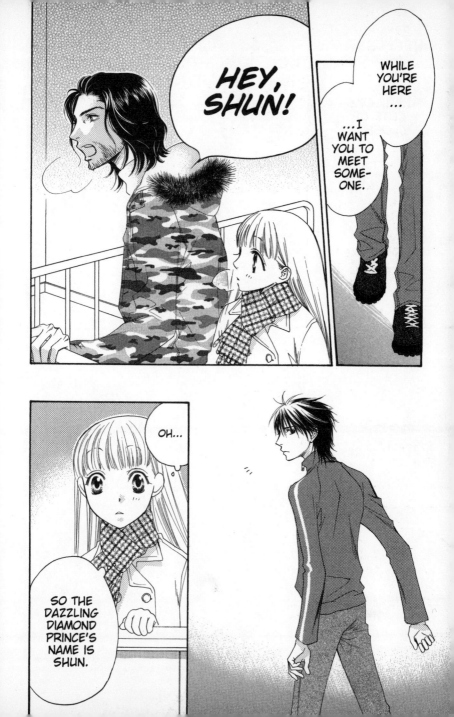

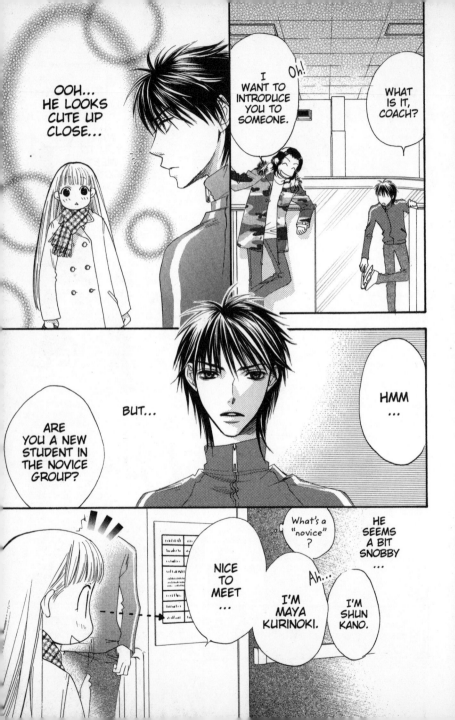

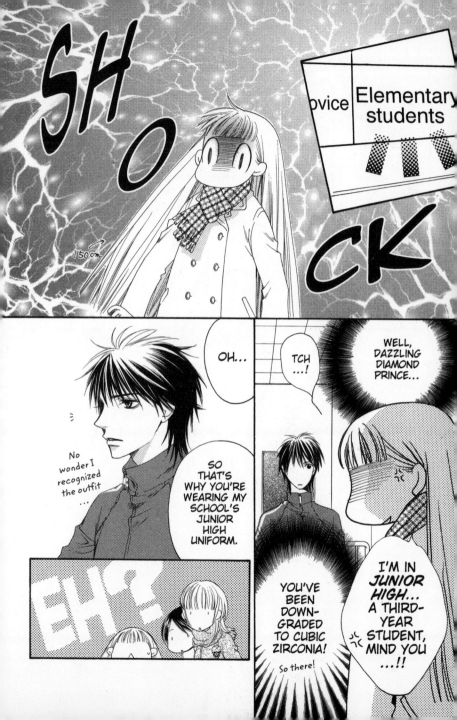

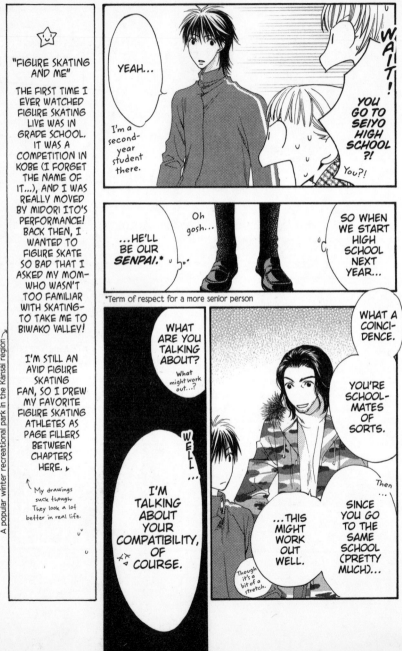

"FIGURE SKATING AND ME"

THE FIRST TIME I EVER WATCHED FIGURE SKATING LIVE WAS IN GRADE SCHOOL. IT WAS A COMPETITION IN KOBE (I FORGET THE NAME OF IT...), AND I WAS REALLY MOVED BY MIDORI ITO'S PERFORMANCE! BACK THEN, I WANTED TO FIGURE SKATE SO BAD THAT I ASKED MY MOM—WHO WASN'T TOO FAMILIAR WITH SKATING—TO TAKE ME TO BIWAKO VALLEY!

I'M STILL AN AVID FIGURE SKATING FAN, SO I DREW MY FAVORITE FIGURE SKATING ATHLETES AS PAGE FILLERS BETWEEN CHAPTERS HERE.

My drawings suck though They look a lot better in real life.

A popular winter recreational park in the Kansai region →

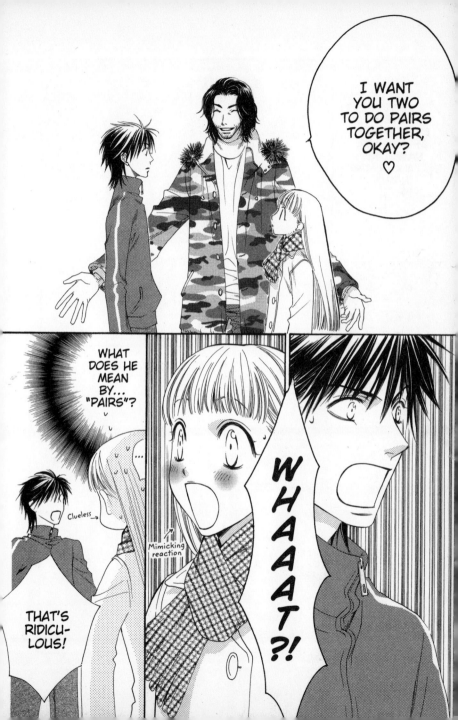

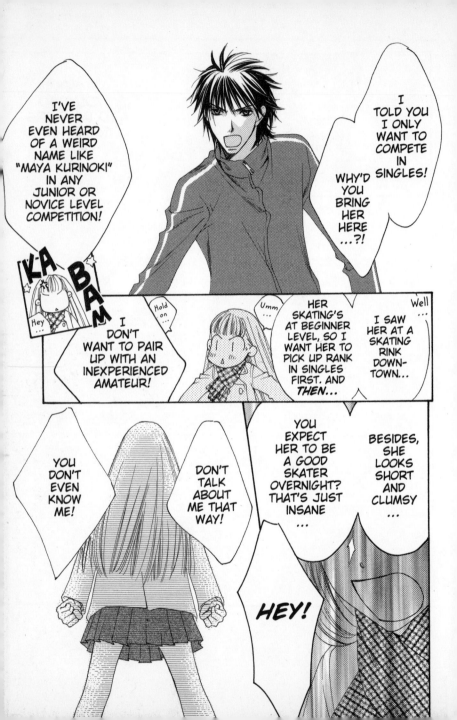

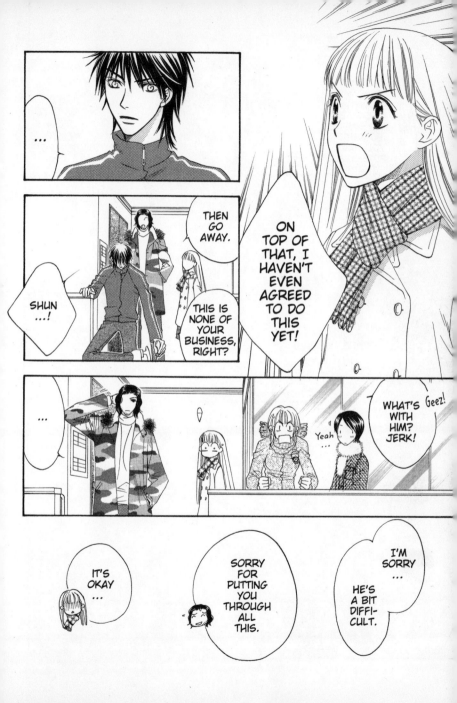

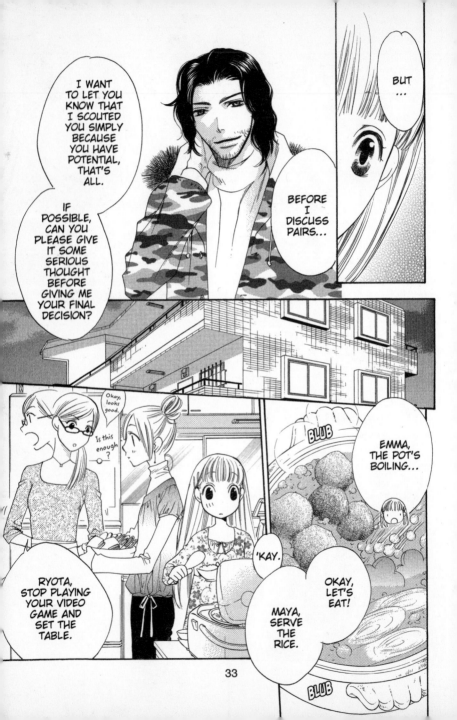

I WANT TO LET YOU KNOW THAT I SCOUTED YOU SIMPLY BECAUSE YOU HAVE POTENTIAL, THAT'S ALL.

IF POSSIBLE, CAN YOU PLEASE GIVE IT SOME SERIOUS THOUGHT BEFORE GIVING ME YOUR FINAL DECISION?

BUT...

BEFORE I DISCUSS PAIRS...

Okay, looks good.

Is this enough?

BLUB

EMMA, THE POT'S BOILING...

RYOTA, STOP PLAYING YOUR VIDEO GAME AND SET THE TABLE.

'KAY.

MAYA, SERVE THE RICE.

OKAY, LET'S EAT!

BLUB

33

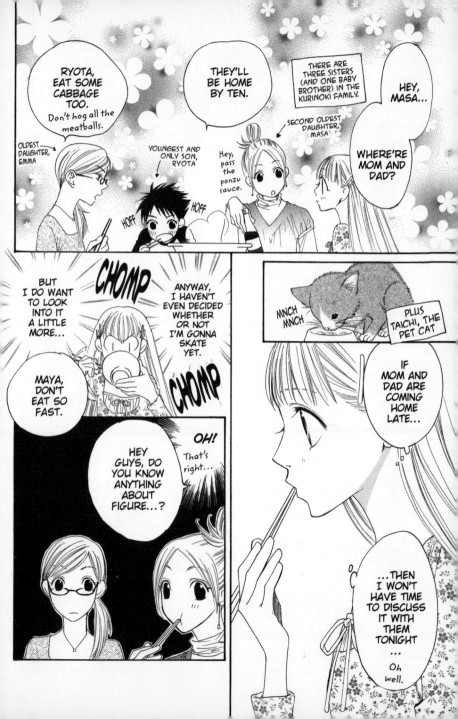

RYOTA, EAT SOME CABBAGE TOO.
Don't hog all the meatballs.

THEY'LL BE HOME BY TEN.

THERE ARE THREE SISTERS (AND ONE BABY BROTHER) IN THE KURINOKI FAMILY.

HEY, MASA...

OLDEST DAUGHTER, EMMA

YOUNGEST AND ONLY SON, RYOTA

SECOND OLDEST DAUGHTER, MASA

Hey, pass the ponzu sauce.

HOFF HOFF

WHERE'RE MOM AND DAD?

BUT I DO WANT TO LOOK INTO IT A LITTLE MORE...

CHOMP

ANYWAY, I HAVEN'T EVEN DECIDED WHETHER OR NOT I'M GONNA SKATE YET.

MAYA, DON'T EAT SO FAST.

CHOMP

OH! That's right...

HEY GUYS, DO YOU KNOW ANYTHING ABOUT FIGURE...?

MNCH MNCH

PLUS TAICHI, THE PET CAT

IF MOM AND DAD ARE COMING HOME LATE...

...THEN I WON'T HAVE TIME TO DISCUSS IT WITH THEM TONIGHT
...
Oh well.

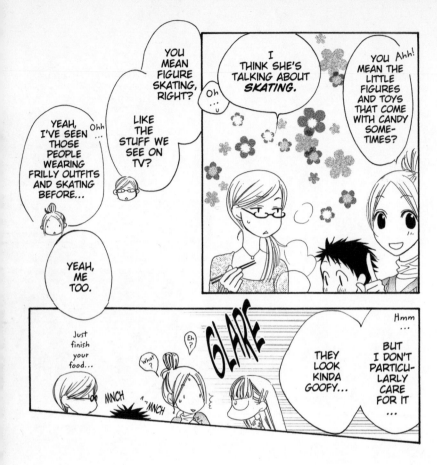

YOU MEAN FIGURE SKATING, RIGHT?

I THINK SHE'S TALKING ABOUT *SKATING.*

Oh

YOU Ahh! MEAN THE LITTLE FIGURES AND TOYS THAT COME WITH CANDY SOME- TIMES?

LIKE THE STUFF WE SEE ON TV?

Ohh ...

YEAH, I'VE SEEN THOSE PEOPLE WEARING FRILLY OUTFITS AND SKATING BEFORE...

YEAH, ME TOO.

Just finish your food...

What?

MNCH

MNCH

Eh?

GLARE

Hmm ...

THEY LOOK KINDA GOOFY...

BUT I DON'T PARTICU- LARLY CARE FOR IT ...

IT WASN'T... GOOFY...

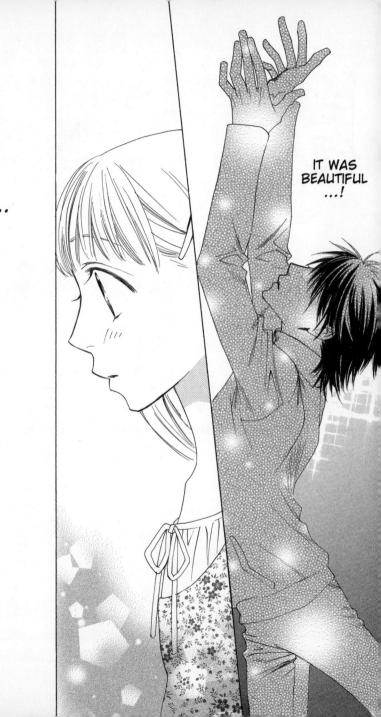

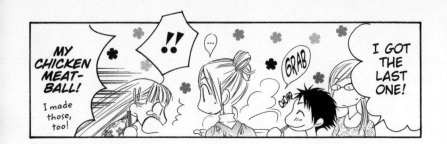

MY CHICKEN MEAT-BALL!

I made those, too!

!!

...

GRAB

CHOMP

I GOT THE LAST ONE!

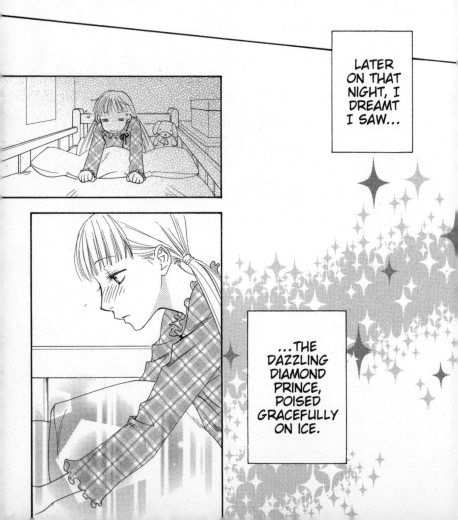

LATER ON THAT NIGHT, I DREAMT I SAW...

...THE DAZZLING DIAMOND PRINCE, POISED GRACEFULLY ON ICE.

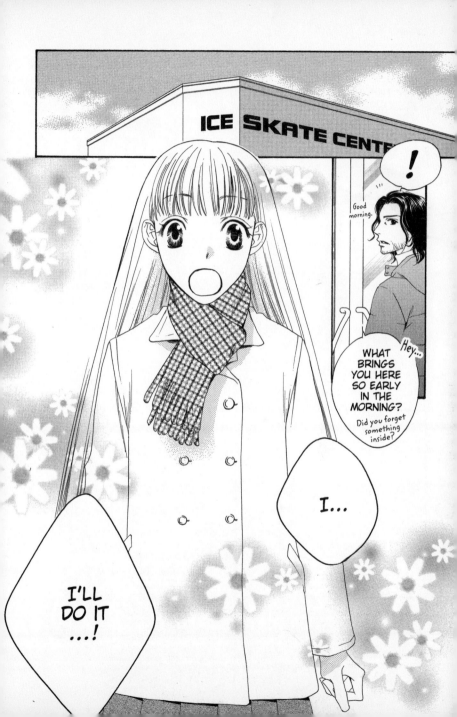

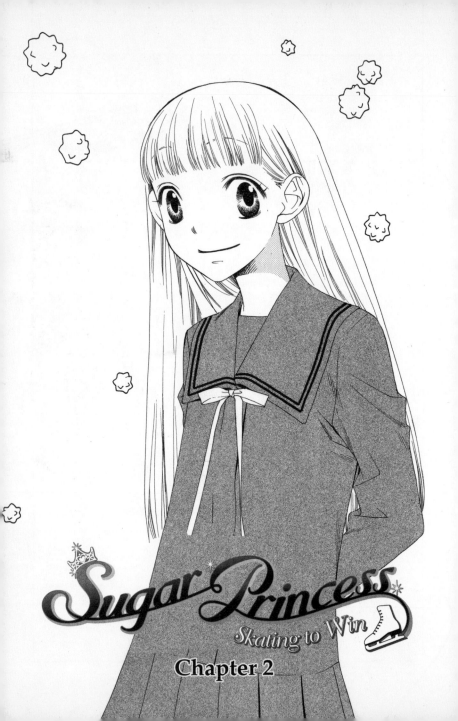

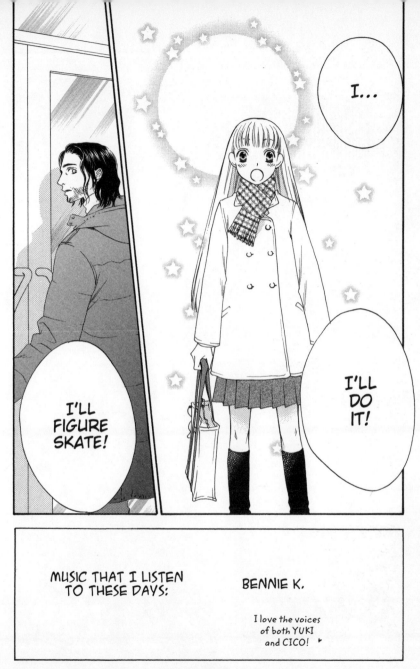

I...

I'LL DO IT!

I'LL FIGURE SKATE!

MUSIC THAT I LISTEN TO THESE DAYS:

BENNIE K.

I love the voices of both YUKI and CICO! ▸

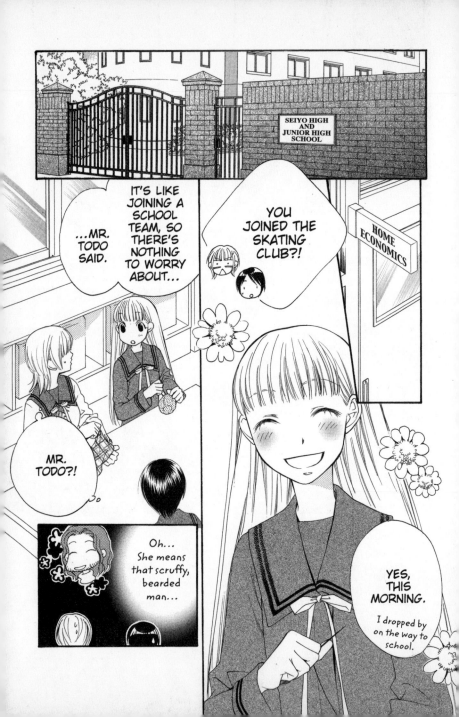

SEIYO HIGH
AND
JUNIOR HIGH
SCHOOL

...MR. TODO SAID.

IT'S LIKE JOINING A SCHOOL TEAM, SO THERE'S NOTHING TO WORRY ABOUT...

YOU JOINED THE SKATING CLUB?!

HOME ECONOMICS

MR. TODO?!

Oh... She means that scruffy, bearded man...

YES, THIS MORNING.

I dropped by on the way to school.

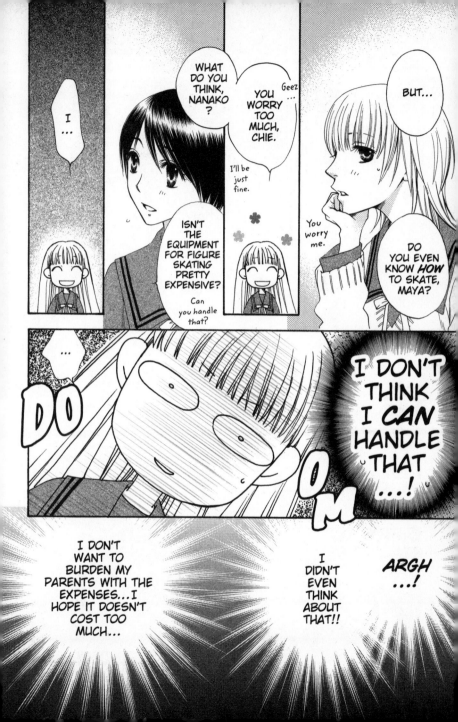

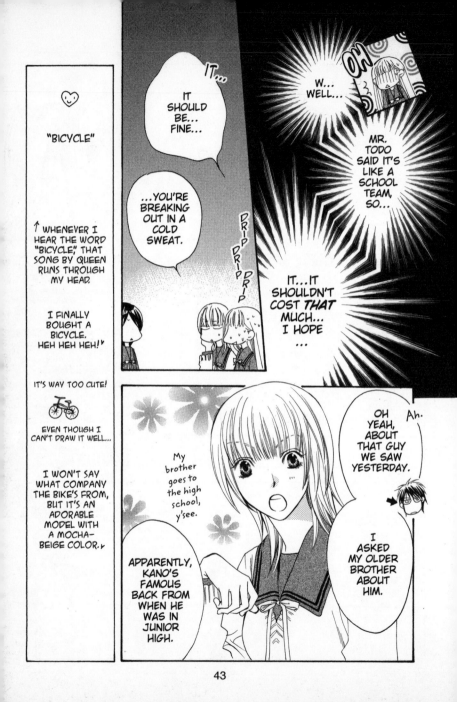

"BICYCLE"

↑ WHENEVER I HEAR THE WORD "BICYCLE," THAT SONG BY QUEEN RUNS THROUGH MY HEAD.

I FINALLY BOUGHT A BICYCLE. HEH HEH HEH!↲

IT'S WAY TOO CUTE!

EVEN THOUGH I CAN'T DRAW IT WELL...

I WON'T SAY WHAT COMPANY THE BIKE'S FROM, BUT IT'S AN ADORABLE MODEL WITH A MOCHA-BEIGE COLOR.↲

IT... IT SHOULD BE... FINE...

...YOU'RE BREAKING OUT IN A COLD SWEAT.

DRIP DRIP DRIP

OH

W... WELL...

MR. TODO SAID IT'S LIKE A SCHOOL TEAM, SO...

IT...IT SHOULDN'T COST THAT MUCH... I HOPE ...

OH YEAH, ABOUT THAT GUY WE SAW YESTERDAY.

Ah.

I ASKED MY OLDER BROTHER ABOUT HIM.

My brother goes to the high school, y'see.

APPARENTLY, KANO'S FAMOUS BACK FROM WHEN HE WAS IN JUNIOR HIGH.

43

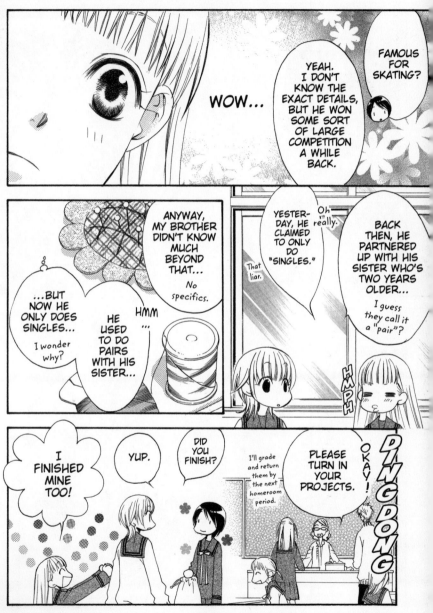

WOW...

FAMOUS FOR SKATING?

YEAH. I DON'T KNOW THE EXACT DETAILS, BUT HE WON SOME SORT OF LARGE COMPETITION A WHILE BACK.

ANYWAY, MY BROTHER DIDN'T KNOW MUCH BEYOND THAT...

No specifics.

YESTER-DAY, HE CLAIMED TO ONLY DO "SINGLES."

Oh really.

That liar.

BACK THEN, HE PARTNERED UP WITH HIS SISTER WHO'S TWO YEARS OLDER...

I guess they call it a "pair"?

...BUT NOW HE ONLY DOES SINGLES...

I wonder why?

HE USED TO DO PAIRS WITH HIS SISTER...

HMM...

HMPH

I FINISHED MINE TOO!

YUP.

DID YOU FINISH?

I'll grade and return them by the next homeroom period.

PLEASE TURN IN YOUR PROJECTS.

OKAY!

DING DONG

44

...

TA DAAA

ISN'T THIS CUTE? I'M GONNA PUT KONPEITO CANDY IN IT. ♡

EH HEH HEH...

It's a tiny candy-bag!

THANKS A LOT, NANAKO.

...CUTE, I GUESS? SORT OF LOOKS LIKE A CRITTER, BUT...ER, NO... I MEAN... IT'S NICE AND FURRY...

IT'S...

Hard to tell if it's cute or not...

YOU'RE QUITE TALENTED AT MAKING *BIZARRE* THINGS...

OH!

I'LL CATCH YOU GUYS BACK AT THE CLASSROOM, OKAY?

I KNOW... THE SIMPLE, SWEET TASTE IS GREAT!

YOUR GRAND-MOTHER'S KONPEITO ALWAYS TASTES WONDER-FUL.

I'll share some with you guys later. ♥

YUP, I GOT SOME YESTER-DAY.

YOUR GRAND-MOTHER SENT MORE KONPEITO TO YOU?

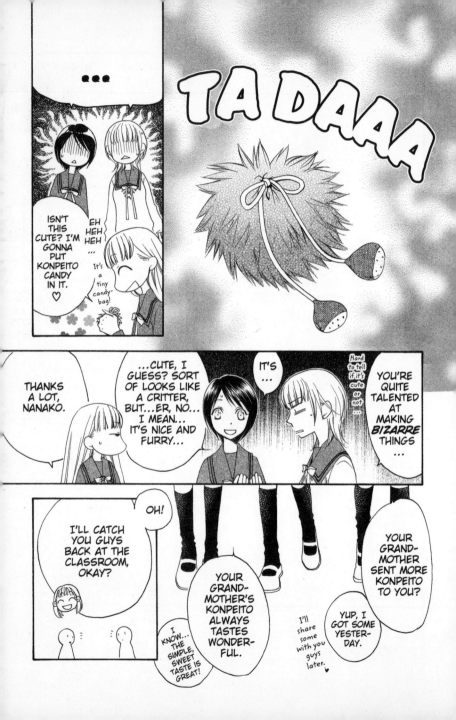

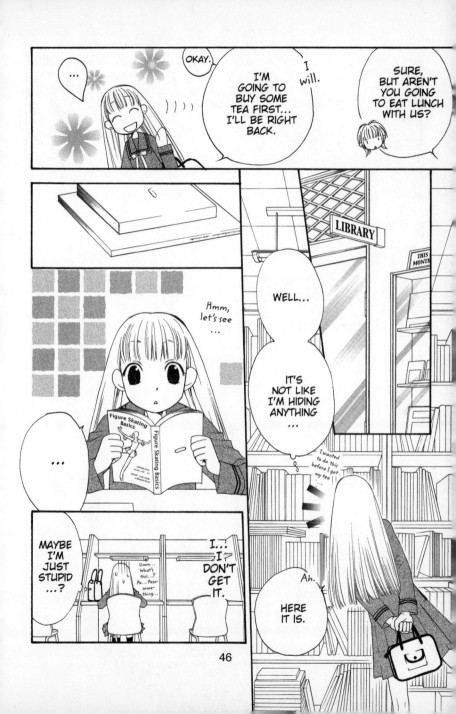

OKAY.

... ✿

I will.

I'M GOING TO BUY SOME TEA FIRST... I'LL BE RIGHT BACK.

SURE, BUT AREN'T YOU GOING TO EAT LUNCH WITH US?

Hmm, let's see ...

LIBRARY

THIS MONTH

WELL...

IT'S NOT LIKE I'M HIDING ANYTHING ...

I wanted to do this before I got my tea...

Figure Skating Basics

...

MAYBE I'M JUST STUPID ...?

Umm... What's this...? Pa... Paso-some-thing...

I... I DON'T GET IT.

Ah.

HERE IT IS.

46

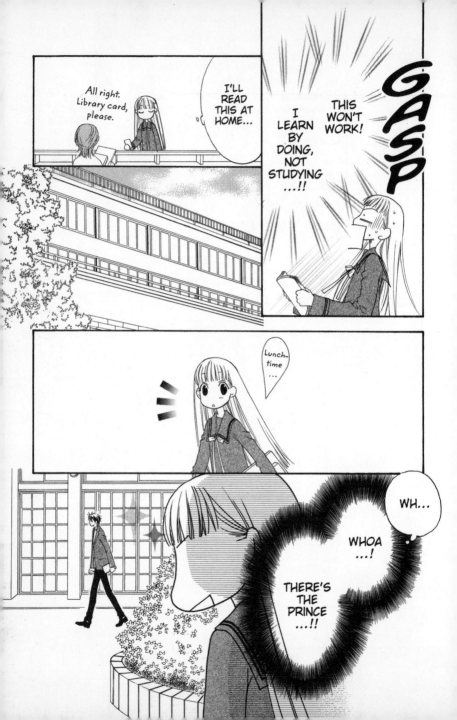

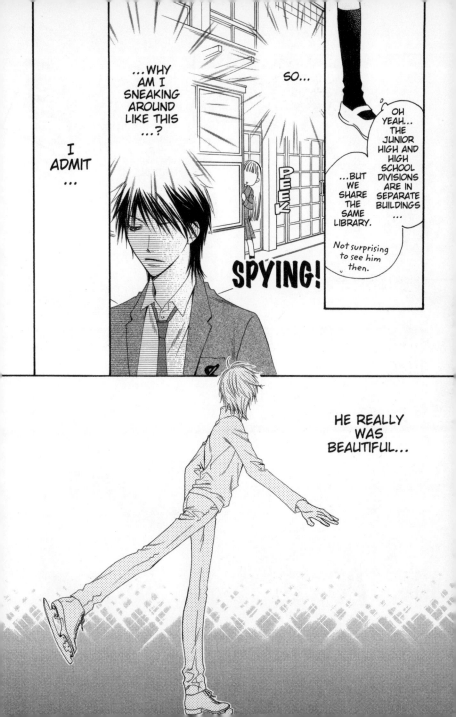

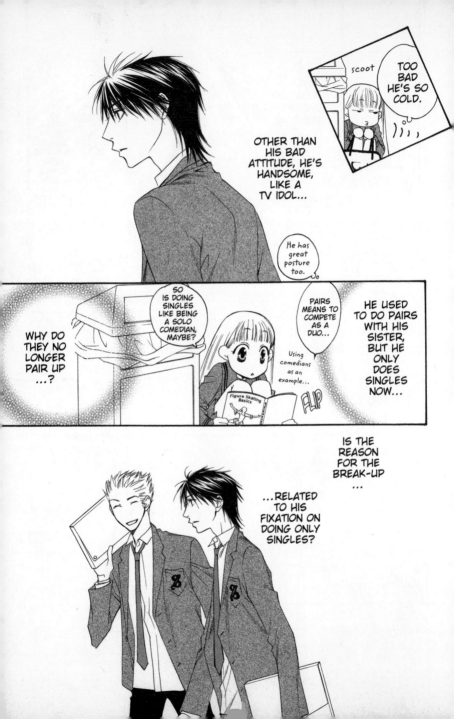

TOO BAD HE'S SO COLD.

scoot

OTHER THAN HIS BAD ATTITUDE, HE'S HANDSOME, LIKE A TV IDOL...

He has great posture too.

WHY DO THEY NO LONGER PAIR UP ...?

IS DOING SINGLES LIKE BEING A SOLO COMEDIAN, MAYBE?

PAIRS MEANS TO COMPETE AS A DUO...

Using comedians as an example...

Figure Skating Basics

FLIP

HE USED TO DO PAIRS WITH HIS SISTER, BUT HE ONLY DOES SINGLES NOW...

IS THE REASON FOR THE BREAK-UP ...

...RELATED TO HIS FIXATION ON DOING ONLY SINGLES?

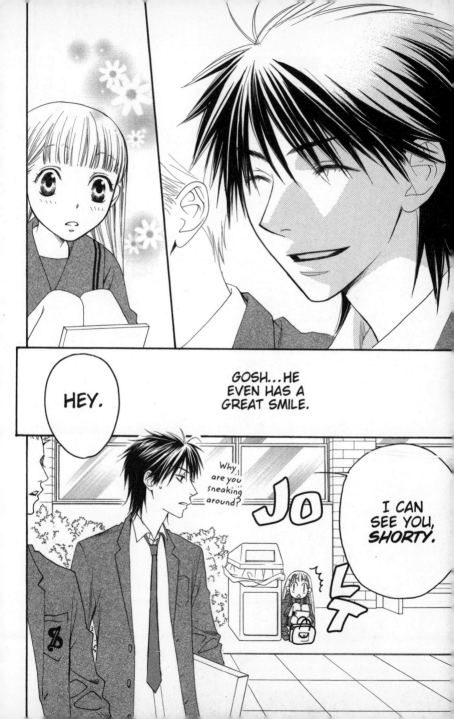

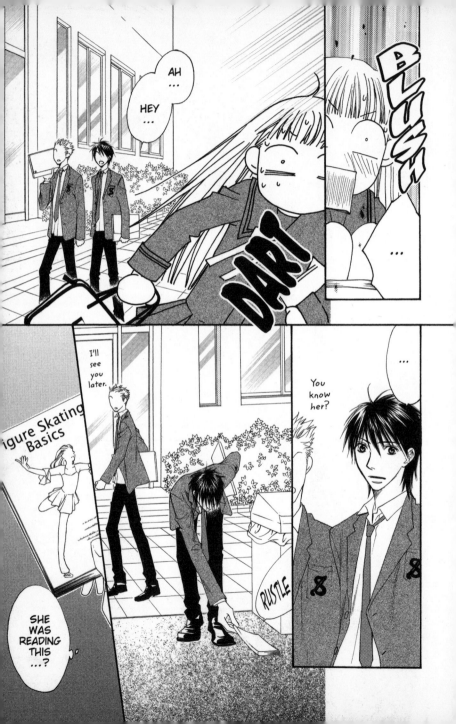

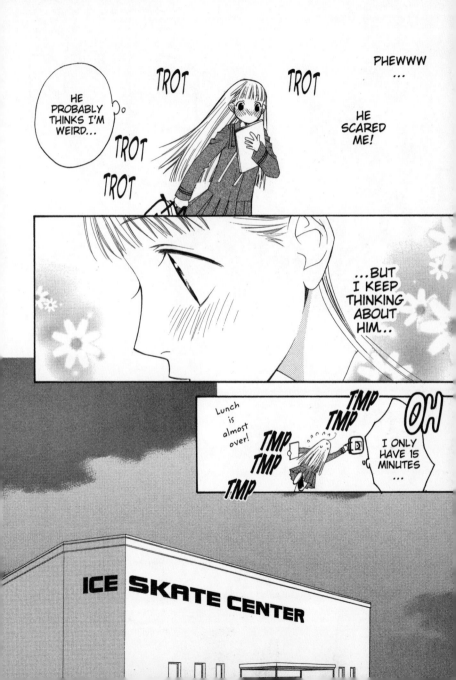

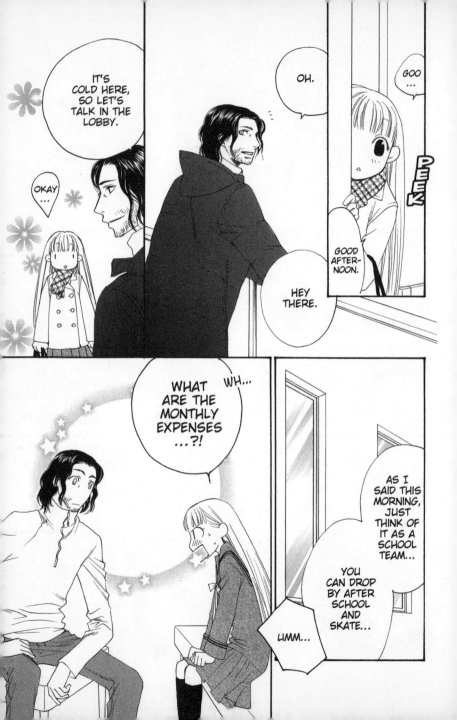

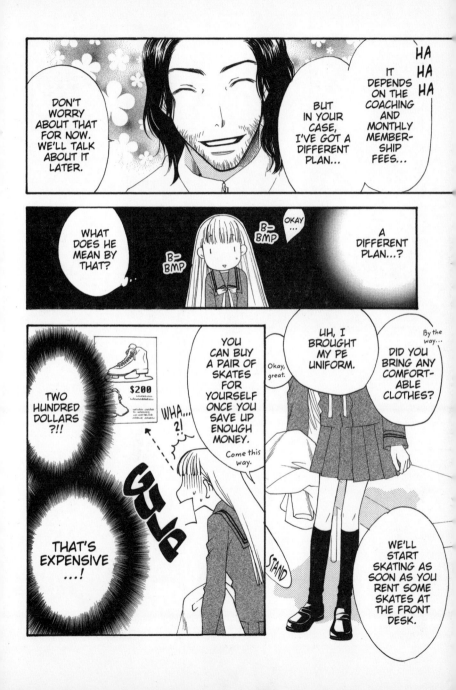

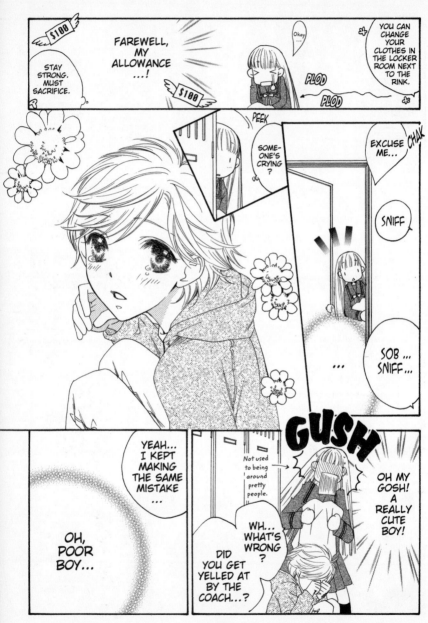

STAY STRONG. MUST SACRIFICE.

FAREWELL, MY ALLOWANCE ...!

$100

$100

Okay

YOU CAN CHANGE YOUR CLOTHES IN THE LOCKER ROOM NEXT TO THE RINK.

PLOD

PLOD

PEEK

SOME-ONE'S CRYING?

EXCUSE ME...

CHAK

SNIFF

...

SOB... SNIFF...

GUSH

YEAH... I KEPT MAKING THE SAME MISTAKE ...

OH, POOR BOY...

Not used to being around pretty people.

WH... WHAT'S WRONG?

DID YOU GET YELLED AT BY THE COACH...?

OH MY GOSH! A REALLY CUTE BOY!

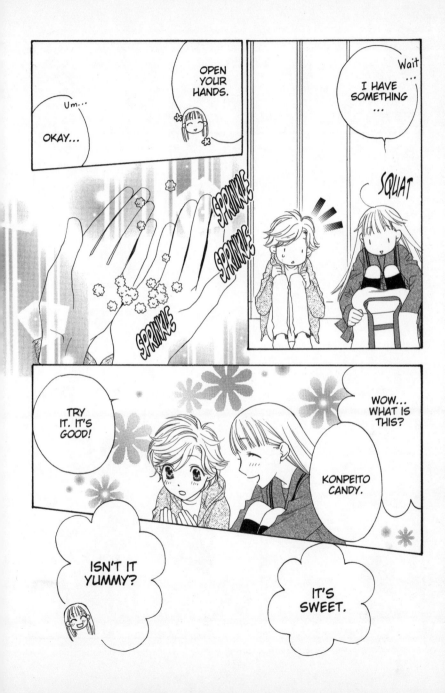

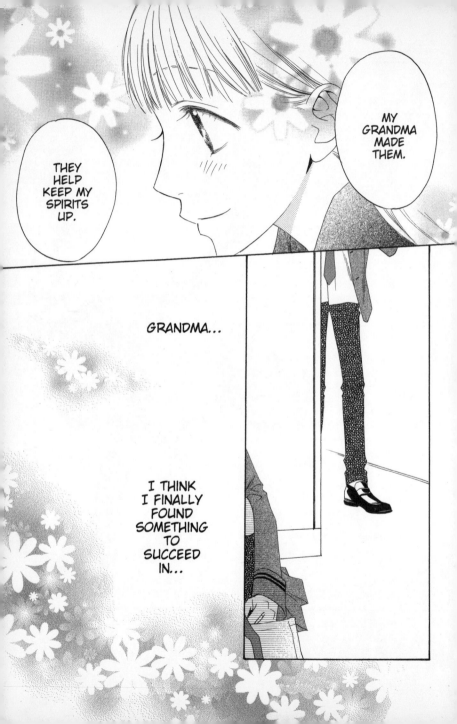

Pairs

Xue SHEN
&
Hongbo ZHAO

My favorite pair. Their
skating is perfect. I got goosebumps when
I saw them at a competition up close.

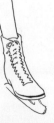

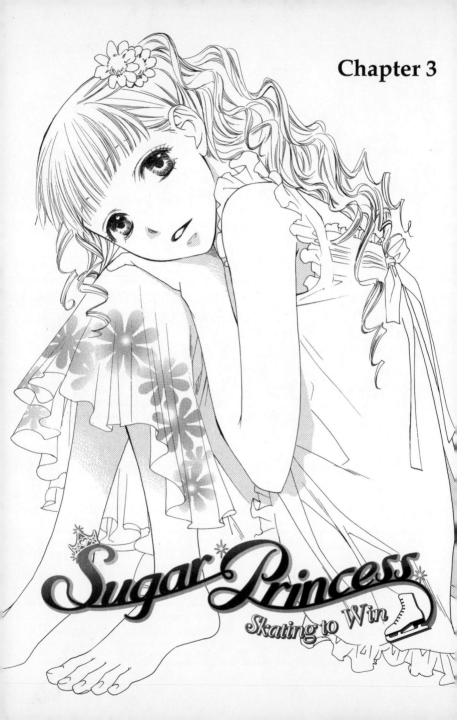

Sugar Princess
Skating to Win

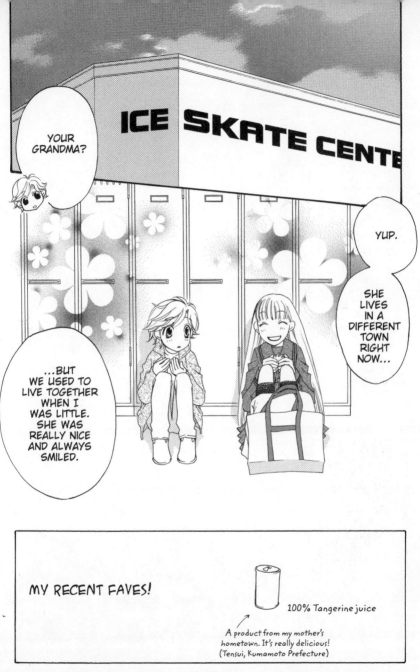

YOUR GRANDMA?

YUP.

SHE LIVES IN A DIFFERENT TOWN RIGHT NOW...

...BUT WE USED TO LIVE TOGETHER WHEN I WAS LITTLE. SHE WAS REALLY NICE AND ALWAYS SMILED.

MY RECENT FAVES!

100% Tangerine juice

A product from my mother's hometown. It's really delicious! (Tensui, Kumamoto Prefecture)

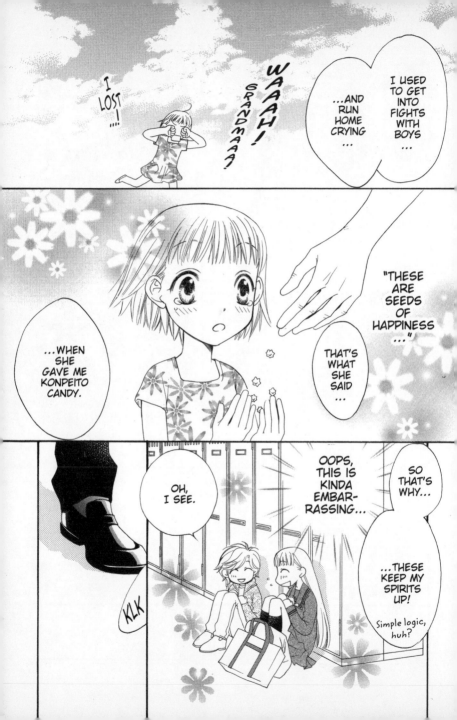

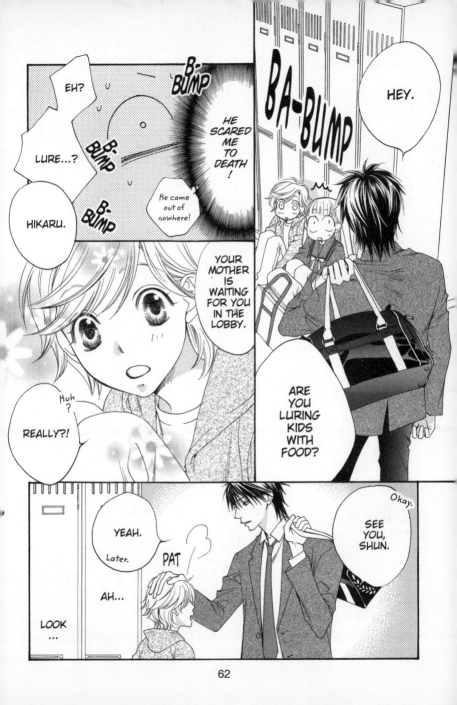

62

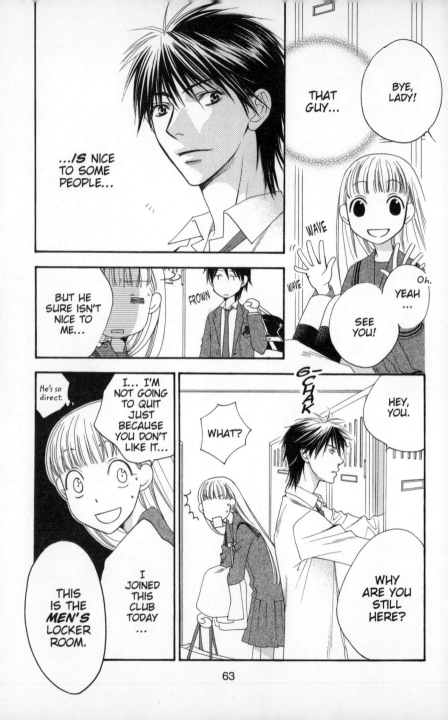

THAT GUY...

BYE, LADY!

...IS NICE TO SOME PEOPLE...

WAVE

WAVE

Oh.

YEAH...

SEE YOU!

BUT HE SURE ISN'T NICE TO ME...

FROWN

He's so direct.

I... I'M NOT GOING TO QUIT JUST BECAUSE YOU DON'T LIKE IT...

WHAT?

G-CHAK

HEY, YOU.

THIS IS THE MEN'S LOCKER ROOM.

I JOINED THIS CLUB TODAY...

WHY ARE YOU STILL HERE?

63

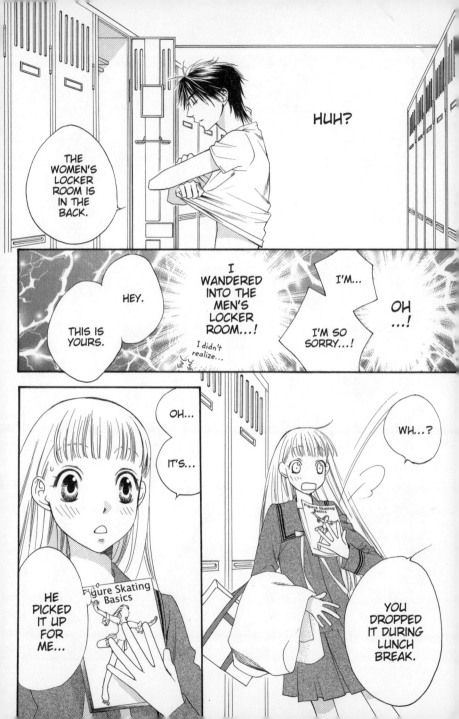

HUH?

THE WOMEN'S LOCKER ROOM IS IN THE BACK.

I WANDERED INTO THE MEN'S LOCKER ROOM...!

I didn't realize...

HEY.

THIS IS YOURS.

I'M...

I'M SO SORRY...!

OH ...!

OH...

IT'S...

WH...?

Figure Skating Basics

HE PICKED IT UP FOR ME...

Figure Skating Basics

YOU DROPPED IT DURING LUNCH BREAK.

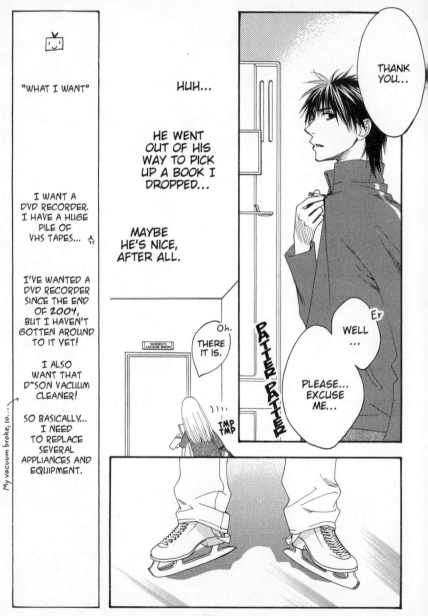

"WHAT I WANT"

I WANT A DVD RECORDER. I HAVE A HUGE PILE OF VHS TAPES...

I'VE WANTED A DVD RECORDER SINCE THE END OF 2004, BUT I HAVEN'T GOTTEN AROUND TO IT YET!

I ALSO WANT THAT D*SON VACUUM CLEANER!

SO BASICALLY... I NEED TO REPLACE SEVERAL APPLIANCES AND EQUIPMENT.

My vacuum broke, so...

HUH...

HE WENT OUT OF HIS WAY TO PICK UP A BOOK I DROPPED...

MAYBE HE'S NICE, AFTER ALL.

THANK YOU...

Er WELL...

PLEASE... EXCUSE ME...

Oh. THERE IT IS.

PATTER PATTER

WOMEN'S LOCKER ROOM

TMP TMP

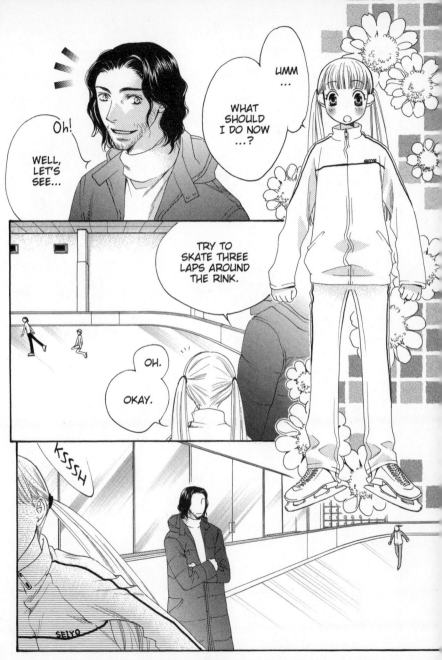

66

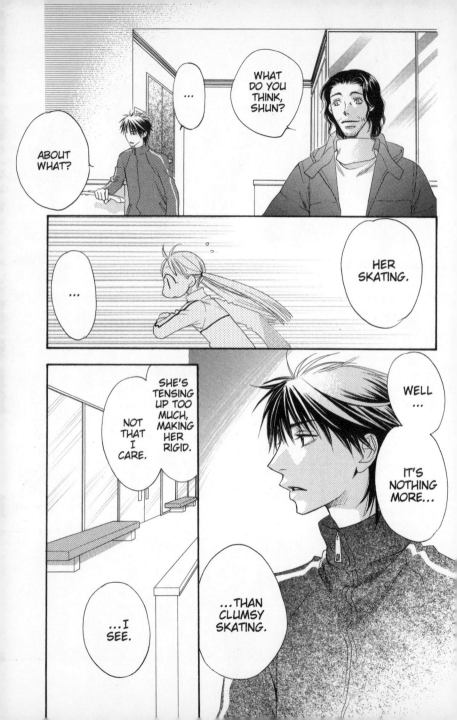

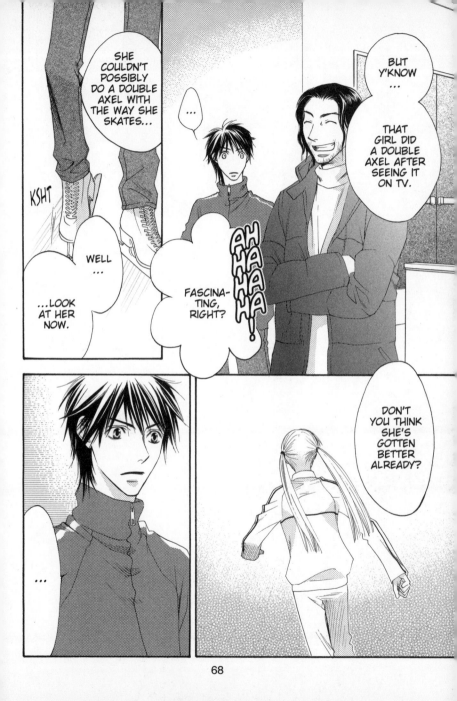

SHE COULDN'T POSSIBLY DO A DOUBLE AXEL WITH THE WAY SHE SKATES...

...

BUT Y'KNOW...

THAT GIRL DID A DOUBLE AXEL AFTER SEEING IT ON TV.

KSHT

WELL...

...LOOK AT HER NOW.

FASCINA-TING, RIGHT?

AH HA HA HA!

DON'T YOU THINK SHE'S GOTTEN BETTER ALREADY?

...

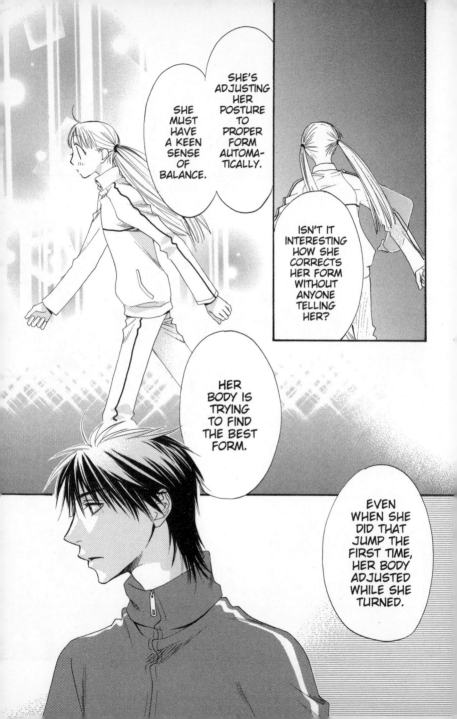

SHE MUST HAVE A KEEN SENSE OF BALANCE.

SHE'S ADJUSTING HER POSTURE TO PROPER FORM AUTOMATICALLY.

ISN'T IT INTERESTING HOW SHE CORRECTS HER FORM WITHOUT ANYONE TELLING HER?

HER BODY IS TRYING TO FIND THE BEST FORM.

EVEN WHEN SHE DID THAT JUMP THE FIRST TIME, HER BODY ADJUSTED WHILE SHE TURNED.

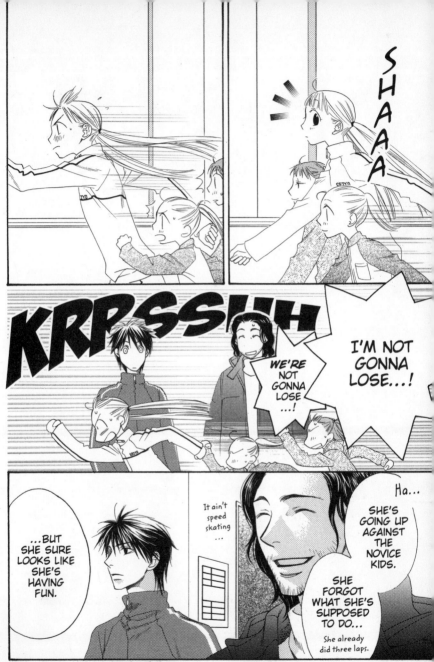

SHAAA

KRPSSHH

WE'RE NOT GONNA LOSE...!

I'M NOT GONNA LOSE...!

Ha...

SHE'S GOING UP AGAINST THE NOVICE KIDS.

It ain't speed skating...

...BUT SHE SURE LOOKS LIKE SHE'S HAVING FUN.

SHE FORGOT WHAT SHE'S SUPPOSED TO DO...

She already did three laps.

*Novice: Class level below Juniors. Ages 9-12 group.

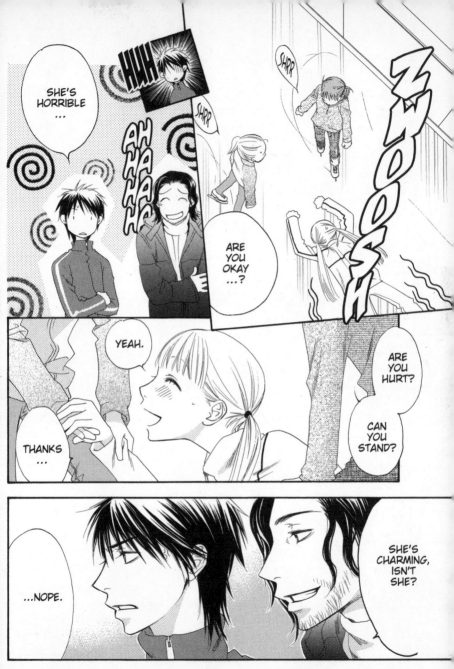

SHE'S HORRIBLE...

HUH

SHRR

SHRR

ZWOOSH

AH HA HA HA

ARE YOU OKAY...?

ARE YOU HURT?

YEAH.

THANKS...

CAN YOU STAND?

...NOPE.

SHE'S CHARMING, ISN'T SHE?

72

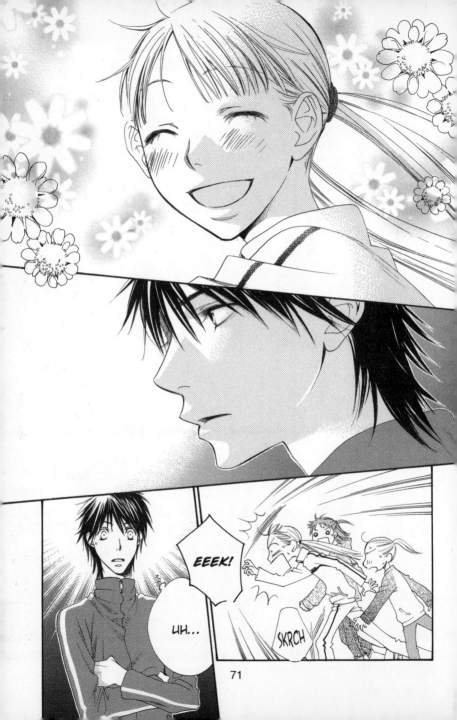

EEEK!

UH...

SKRCH

71

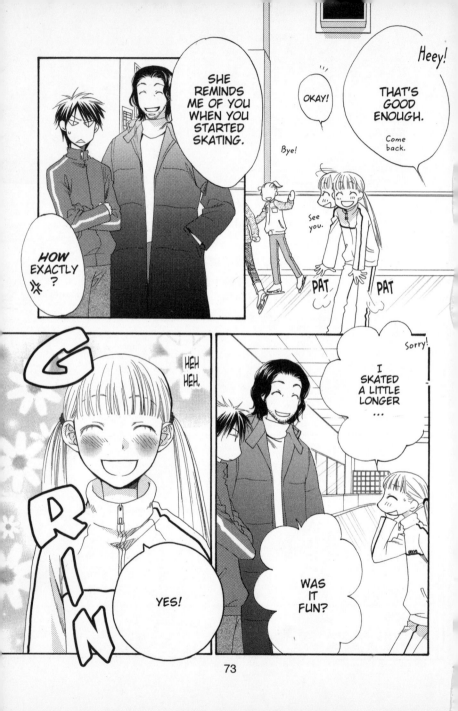

SHE REMINDS ME OF YOU WHEN YOU STARTED SKATING.

HOW EXACTLY ※ ?

Heey!

OKAY!

THAT'S GOOD ENOUGH.

Come back.

Bye!

See you.

PAT

PAT

HEH HEH,

GRIN

YES!

Sorry!

I SKATED A LITTLE LONGER ...

WAS IT FUN?

73

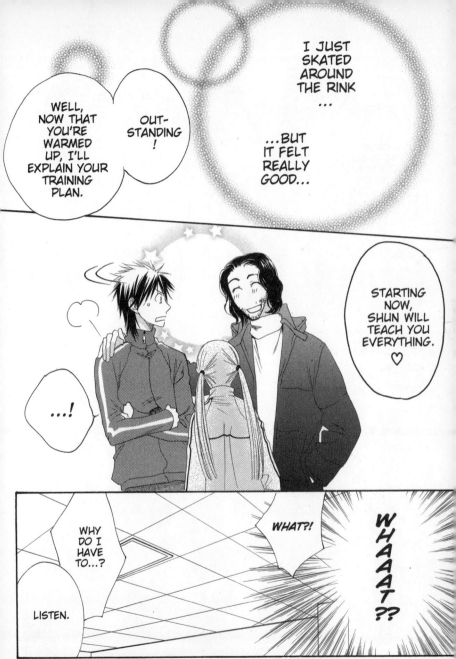

I JUST SKATED AROUND THE RINK ...

...BUT IT FELT REALLY GOOD...

WELL, NOW THAT YOU'RE WARMED UP, I'LL EXPLAIN YOUR TRAINING PLAN.

OUT-STANDING!

STARTING NOW, SHUN WILL TEACH YOU EVERYTHING. ♡

...!

WHY DO I HAVE TO...?

WHAT?!

WHAAAT??

LISTEN.

*Badge test - Test to determine the most appropriate skating level/rank. There are eight levels.

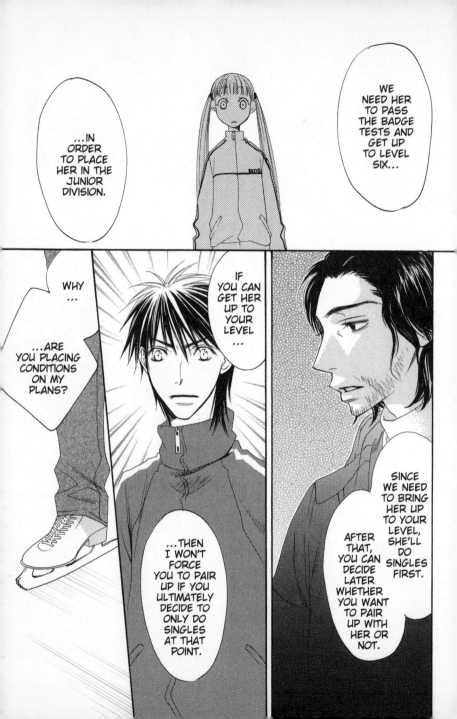

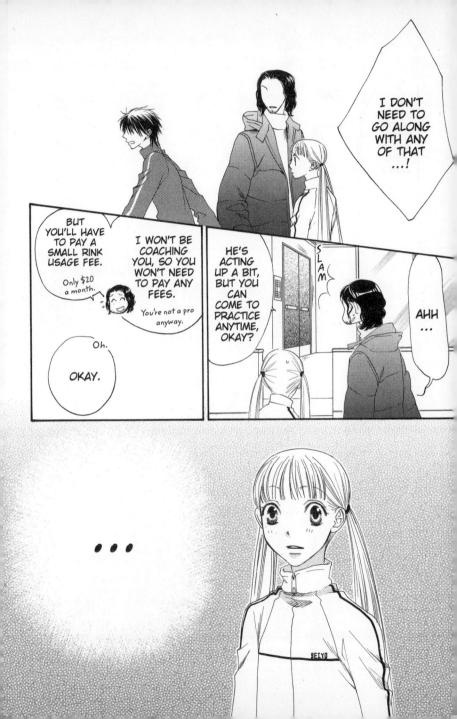

I DON'T NEED TO GO ALONG WITH ANY OF THAT ...!

BUT YOU'LL HAVE TO PAY A SMALL RINK USAGE FEE.

Only $20 a month.

I WON'T BE COACHING YOU, SO YOU WON'T NEED TO PAY ANY FEES.

You're not a pro anyway.

Oh.

OKAY.

HE'S ACTING UP A BIT, BUT YOU CAN COME TO PRACTICE ANYTIME, OKAY?

SLAM

AHH ...

• • •

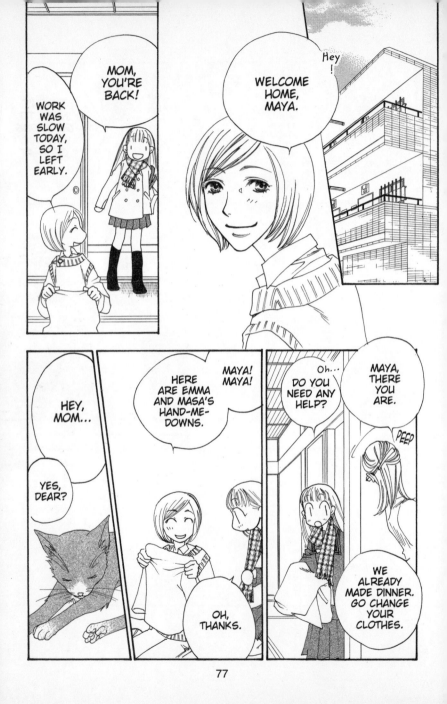

77

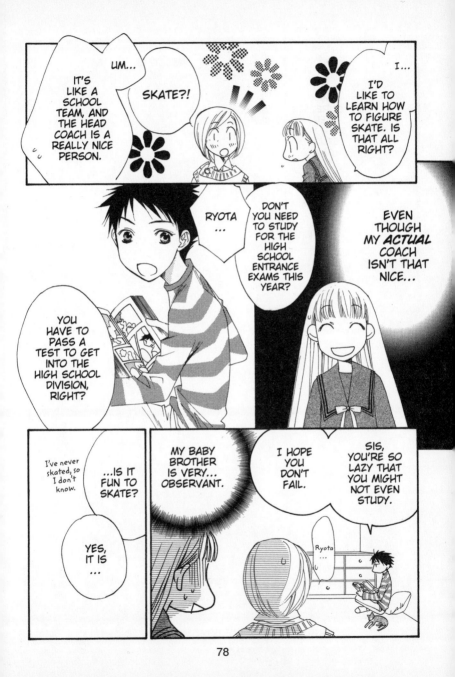

UM...

SKATE?!

IT'S LIKE A SCHOOL TEAM, AND THE HEAD COACH IS A REALLY NICE PERSON.

I...

I'D LIKE TO LEARN HOW TO FIGURE SKATE. IS THAT ALL RIGHT?

RYOTA...

DON'T YOU NEED TO STUDY FOR THE HIGH SCHOOL ENTRANCE EXAMS THIS YEAR?

EVEN THOUGH MY *ACTUAL* COACH ISN'T THAT NICE...

YOU HAVE TO PASS A TEST TO GET INTO THE HIGH SCHOOL DIVISION, RIGHT?

I've never skated, so I don't know.

...IS IT FUN TO SKATE?

MY BABY BROTHER IS VERY... OBSERVANT.

I HOPE YOU DON'T FAIL.

SIS, YOU'RE SO LAZY THAT YOU MIGHT NOT EVEN STUDY.

YES, IT IS...

Ryota...

78

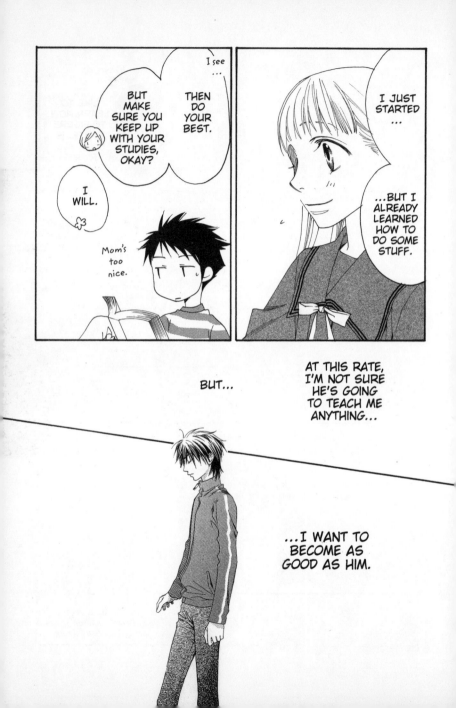

Dance

Marina ANISSINA
&
Gwendal PEIZERAT

*A couple with everything
a girl dreams about! So graceful
and wonderful! I love them...!*

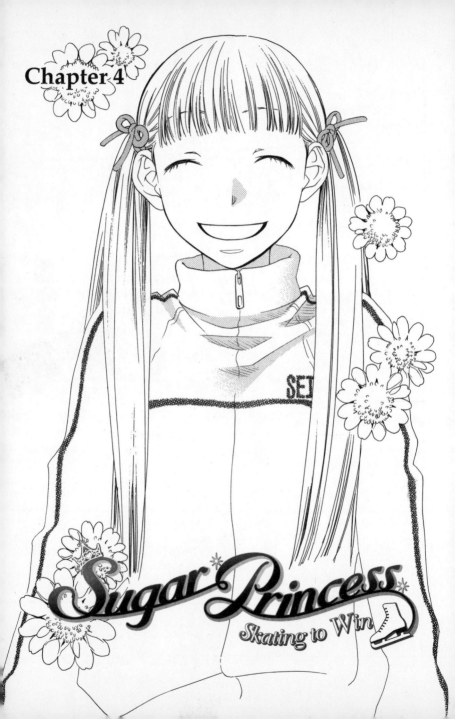

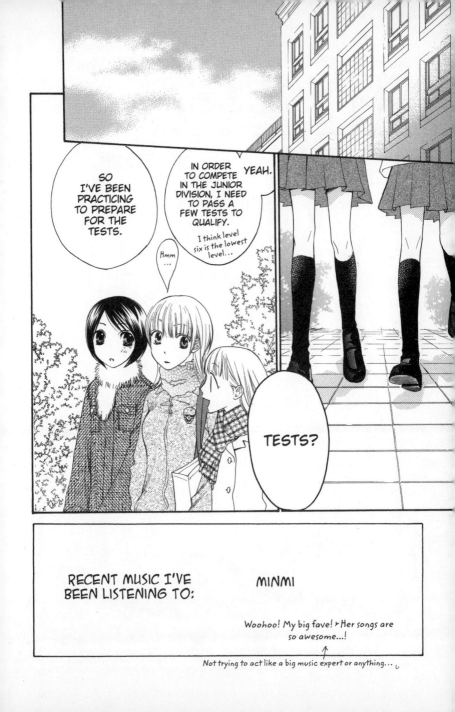

SO I'VE BEEN PRACTICING TO PREPARE FOR THE TESTS.

Hmm...

IN ORDER TO COMPETE IN THE JUNIOR DIVISION, I NEED TO PASS A FEW TESTS TO QUALIFY.

YEAH.

I think level six is the lowest level...

TESTS?

RECENT MUSIC I'VE BEEN LISTENING TO:

MINMI

Woohoo! My big fave! ♪ Her songs are so awesome...!

Not trying to act like a big music expert or anything...

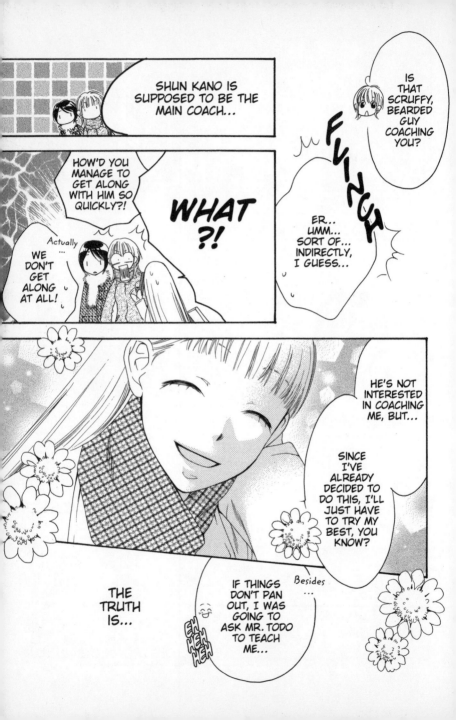

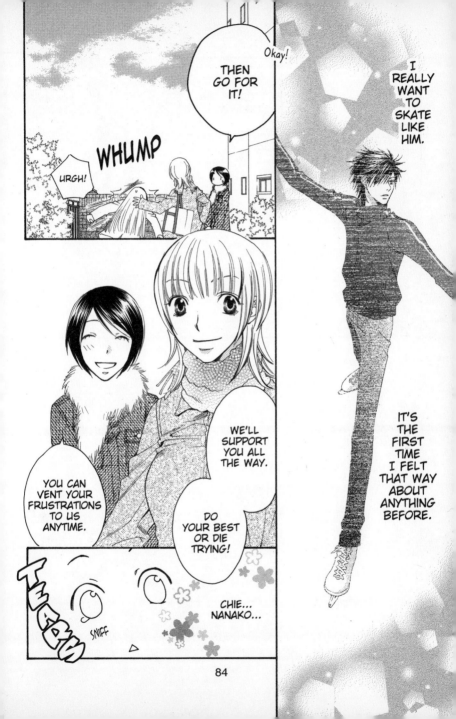

THEN GO FOR IT!

Okay!

I REALLY WANT TO SKATE LIKE HIM.

WHUMP

URGH!

WE'LL SUPPORT YOU ALL THE WAY.

YOU CAN VENT YOUR FRUSTRATIONS TO US ANYTIME.

DO YOUR BEST OR DIE TRYING!

IT'S THE FIRST TIME I FELT THAT WAY ABOUT ANYTHING BEFORE.

TEAM

SNIFF

CHIE... NANAKO...

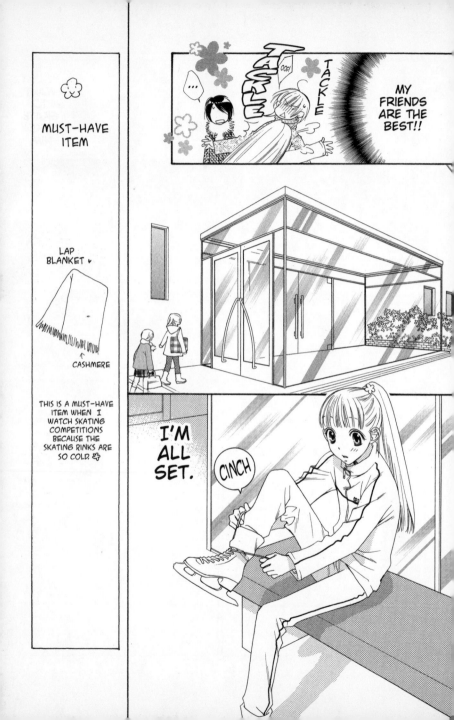

MY FRIENDS ARE THE BEST!!

OOF!

TACKLE

...

MUST-HAVE ITEM

LAP BLANKET ↵

↑ CASHMERE

THIS IS A MUST-HAVE ITEM WHEN I WATCH SKATING COMPETITIONS BECAUSE THE SKATING RINKS ARE SO COLD. ❧

I'M ALL SET.

CINCH

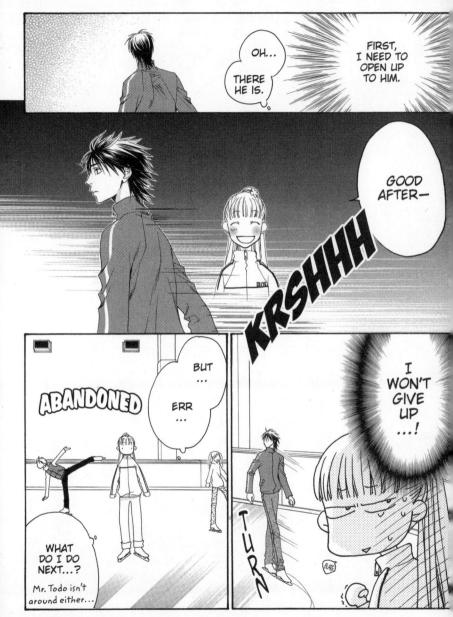

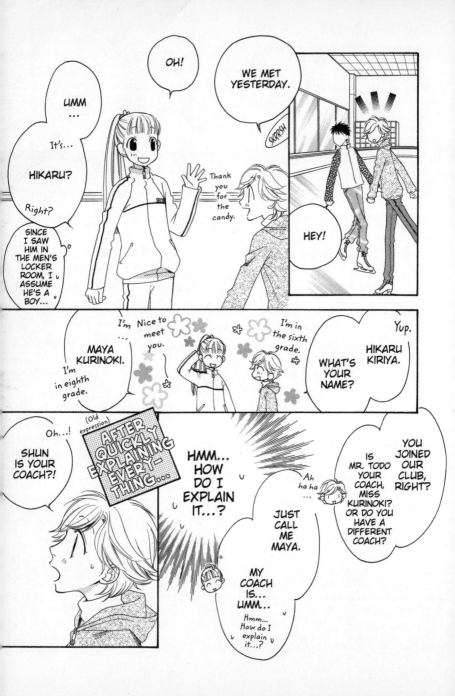

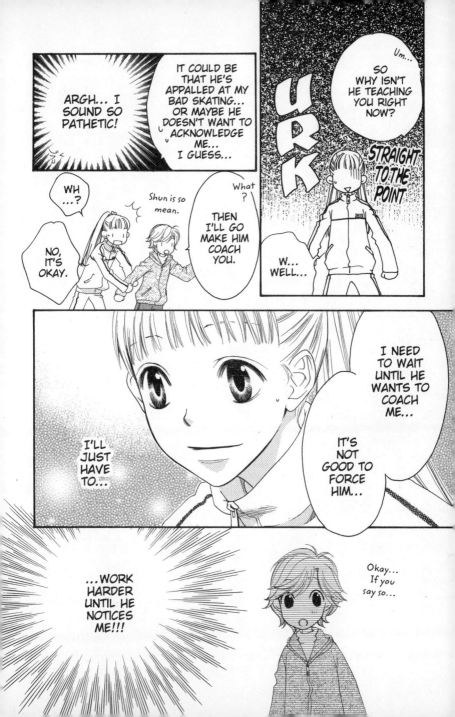

ARGH... I SOUND SO PATHETIC!

IT COULD BE THAT HE'S APPALLED AT MY BAD SKATING... OR MAYBE HE DOESN'T WANT TO ACKNOWLEDGE ME... I GUESS...

Um... SO WHY ISN'T HE TEACHING YOU RIGHT NOW?

URK

STRAIGHT TO THE POINT

WH ...?

Shun is so mean.

What ?

THEN I'LL GO MAKE HIM COACH YOU.

NO, IT'S OKAY.

W... WELL...

I NEED TO WAIT UNTIL HE WANTS TO COACH ME...

IT'S NOT GOOD TO FORCE HIM...

I'LL JUST HAVE TO...

...WORK HARDER UNTIL HE NOTICES ME!!!

Okay... If you say so...

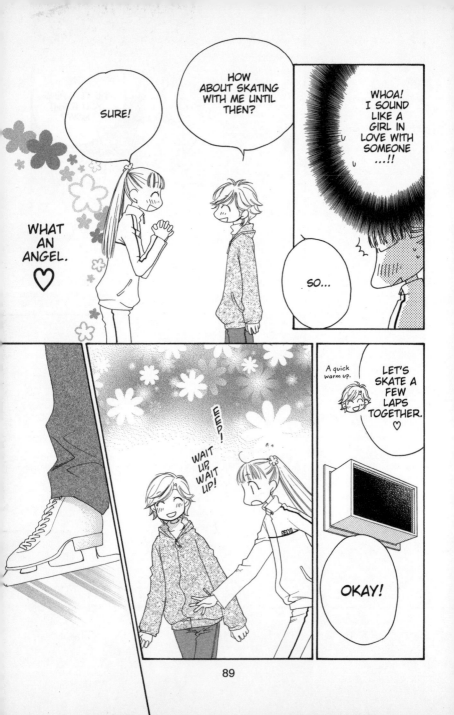

SURE!

HOW ABOUT SKATING WITH ME UNTIL THEN?

WHOA! I SOUND LIKE A GIRL IN LOVE WITH SOMEONE ...!!

WHAT AN ANGEL. ♡

SO...

LET'S SKATE A FEW LAPS TOGETHER. ♡

A quick warm up.

EEP!

WAIT UP WAIT UP!

OKAY!

89

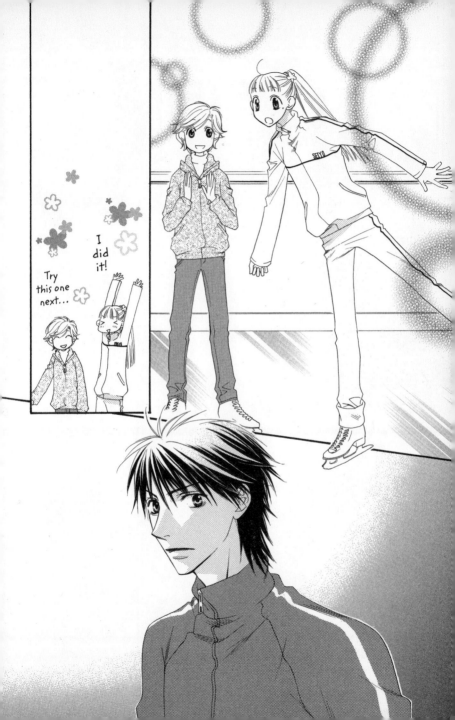

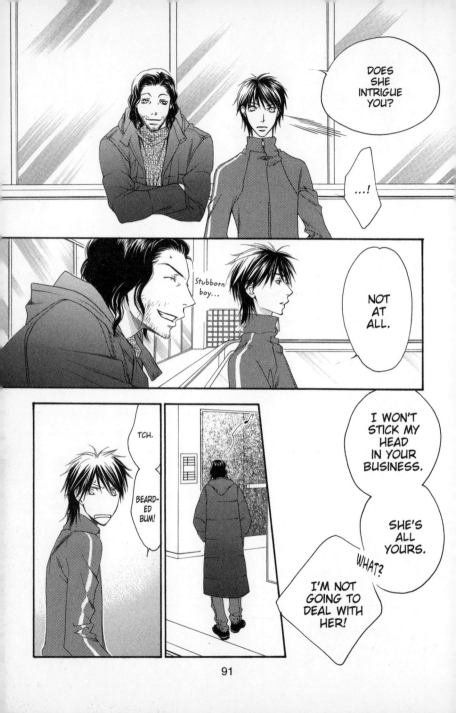

91

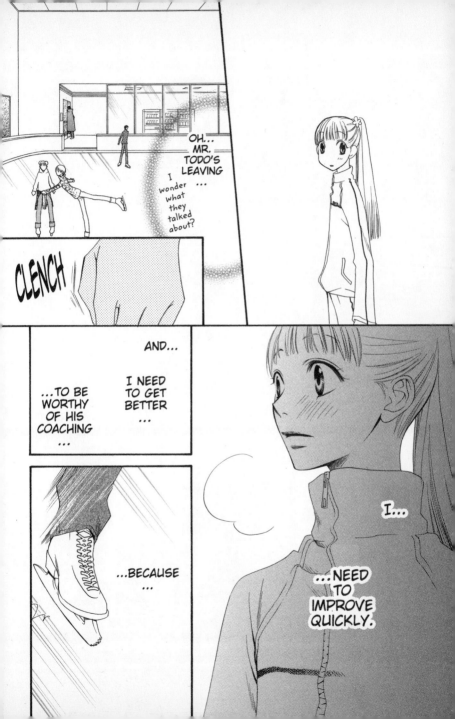

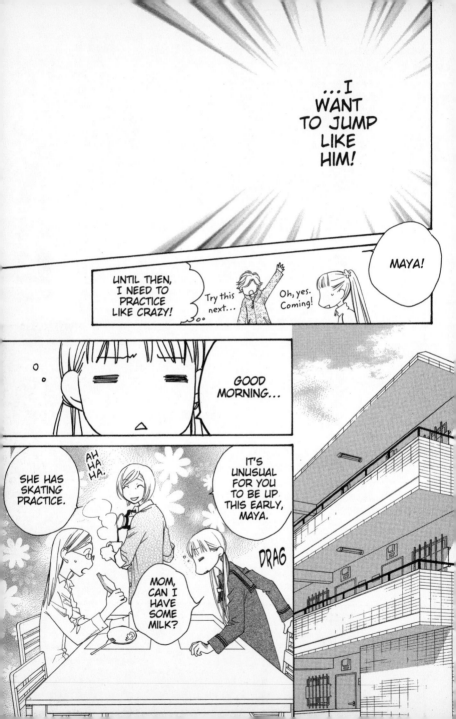

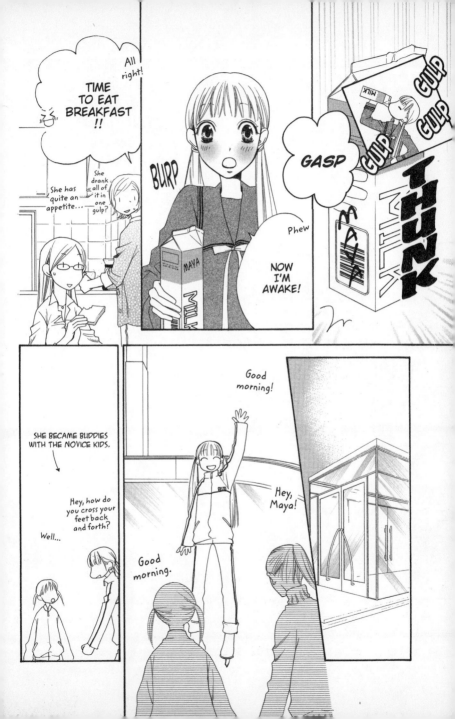

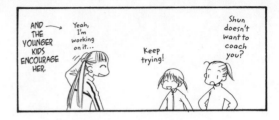

AND THE YOUNGER KIDS ENCOURAGE HER.

→ Yeah, I'm working on it...

Keep trying!

Shun doesn't want to coach you?

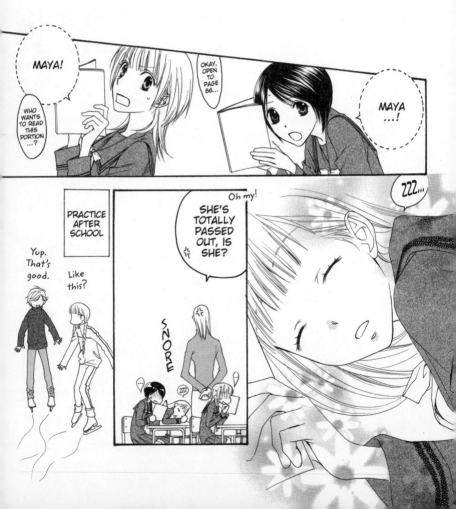

MAYA!

WHO WANTS TO READ THIS PORTION...?

OKAY, OPEN TO PAGE 86...

MAYA...!

PRACTICE AFTER SCHOOL

Yup. That's good.

Like this?

Oh my!

SHE'S TOTALLY PASSED OUT, IS SHE?

SNORE

ZZZ...

ZZZ,,,,

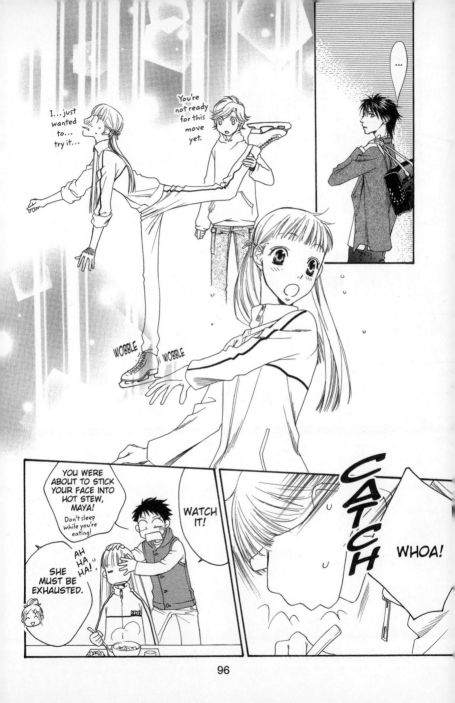

96

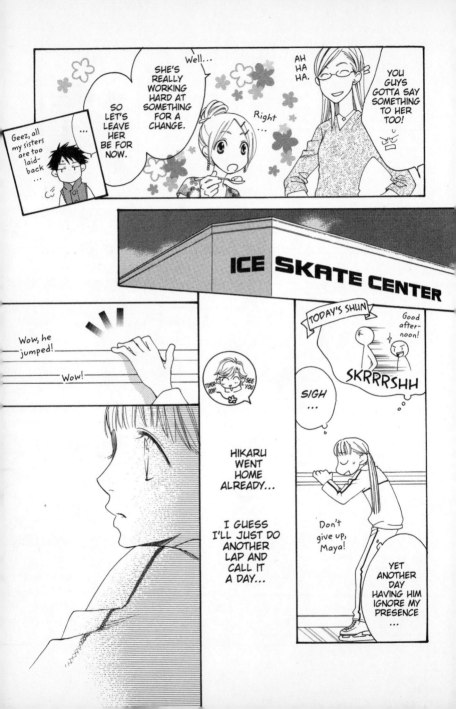

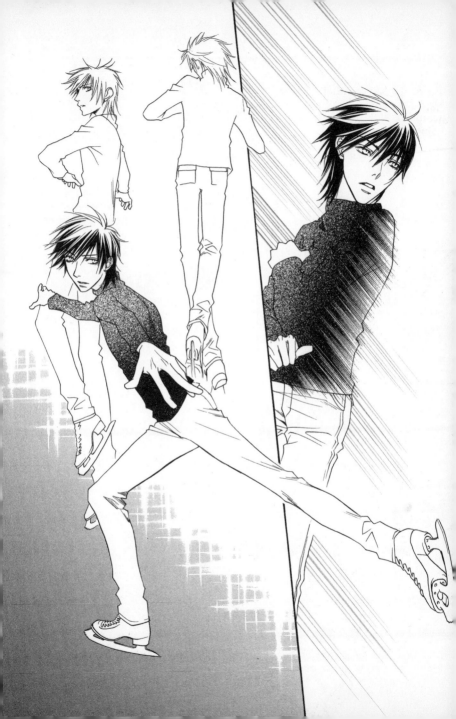

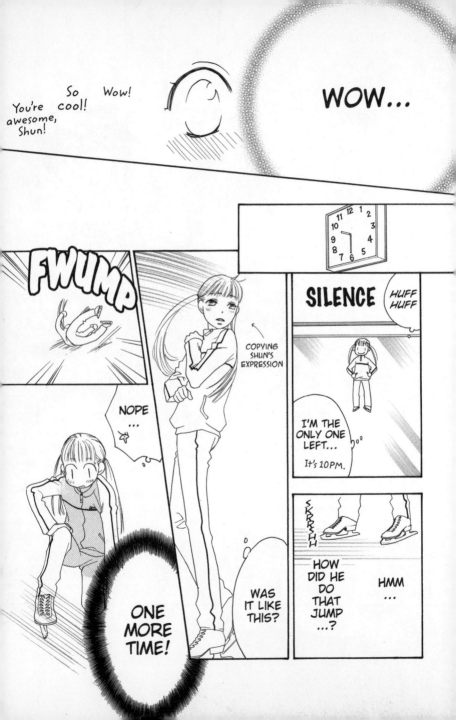

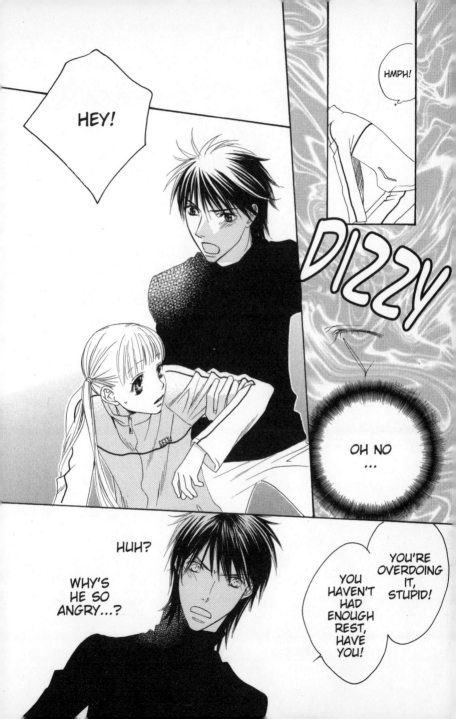

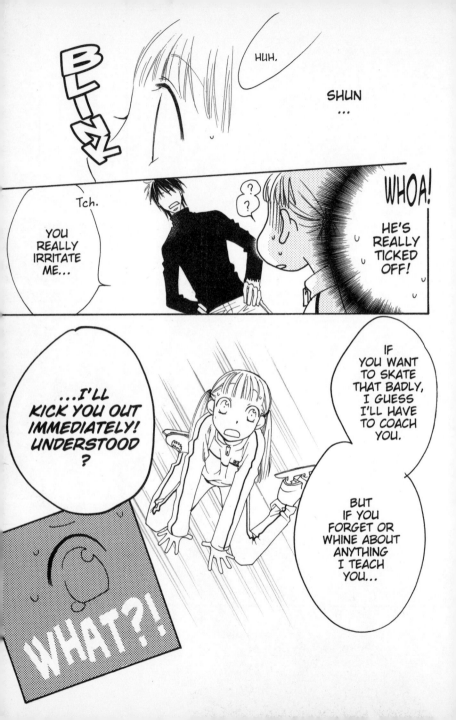

Dance

They are a very fresh and daring couple. I'll never forget their performance to Michael Jackson's music! I love them!

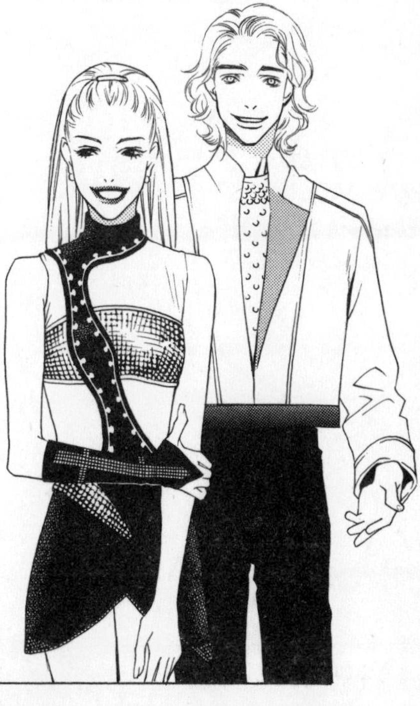

Shae-Lynn BOURNE
&
Victor KRAATZ

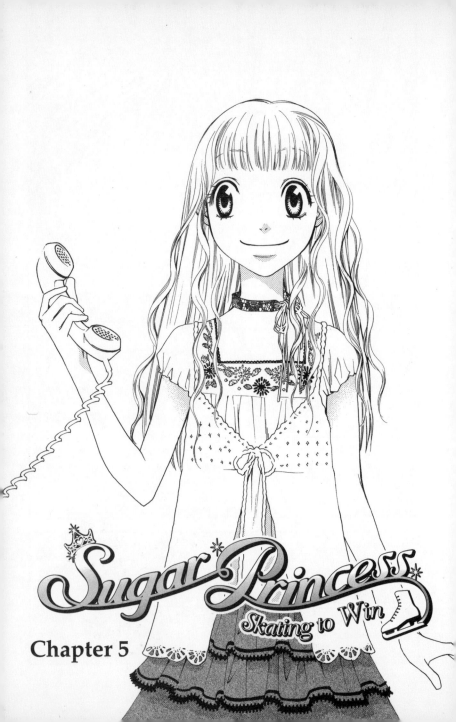

Sugar Princess
Skating to Win

Chapter 5

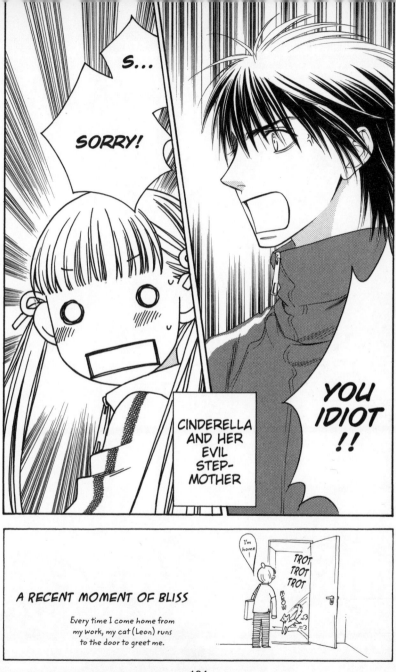

104

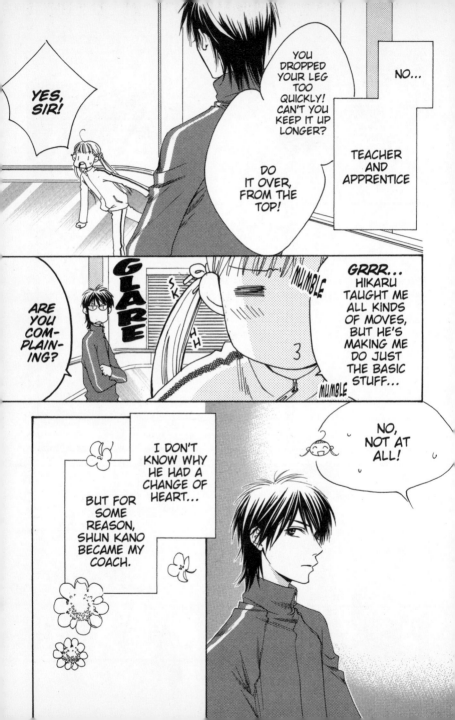

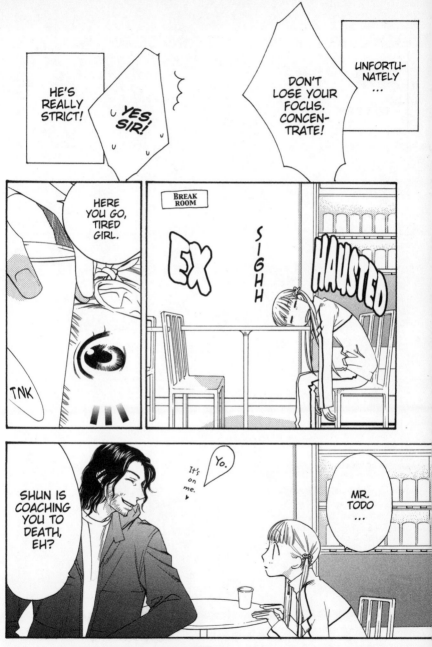

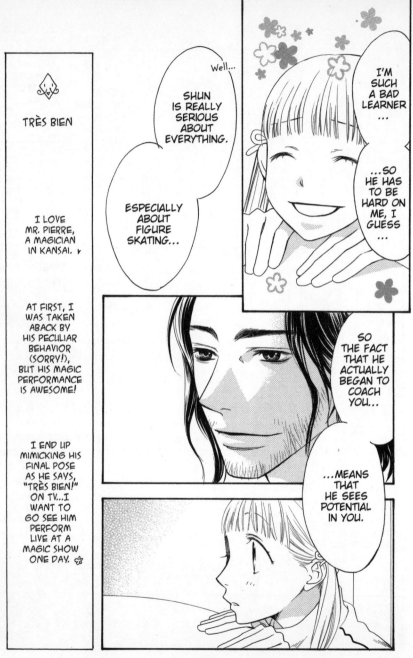

TRÈS BIEN

I LOVE MR. PIERRE, A MAGICIAN IN KANSAI. ▸

AT FIRST, I WAS TAKEN ABACK BY HIS PECULIAR BEHAVIOR (SORRY!), BUT HIS MAGIC PERFORMANCE IS AWESOME!

I END UP MIMICKING HIS FINAL POSE AS HE SAYS, "TRÈS BIEN!" ON TV...I WANT TO GO SEE HIM PERFORM LIVE AT A MAGIC SHOW ONE DAY. ✿

Well...

SHUN IS REALLY SERIOUS ABOUT EVERYTHING.

ESPECIALLY ABOUT FIGURE SKATING...

I'M SUCH A BAD LEARNER...

...SO HE HAS TO BE HARD ON ME, I GUESS...

SO THE FACT THAT HE ACTUALLY BEGAN TO COACH YOU...

...MEANS THAT HE SEES POTENTIAL IN YOU.

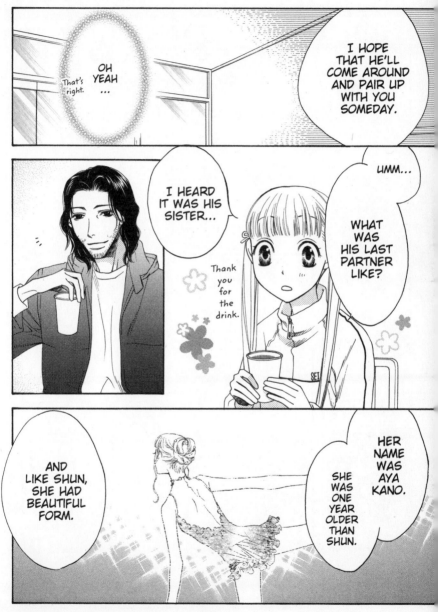

I HOPE THAT HE'LL COME AROUND AND PAIR UP WITH YOU SOMEDAY.

OH YEAH ...

That's right.

UMM...

WHAT WAS HIS LAST PARTNER LIKE?

I HEARD IT WAS HIS SISTER...

Thank you for the drink.

HER NAME WAS AYA KANO.

SHE WAS ONE YEAR OLDER THAN SHUN.

AND LIKE SHUN, SHE HAD BEAUTIFUL FORM.

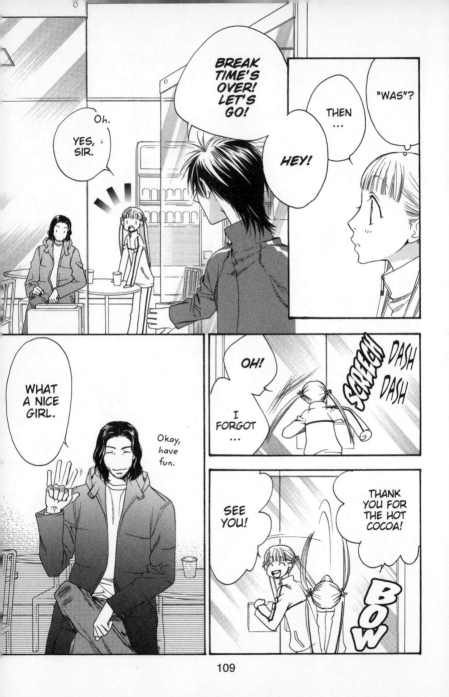

109

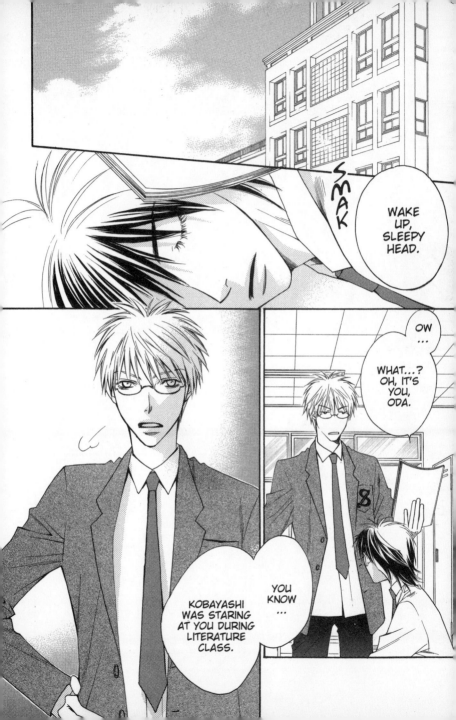

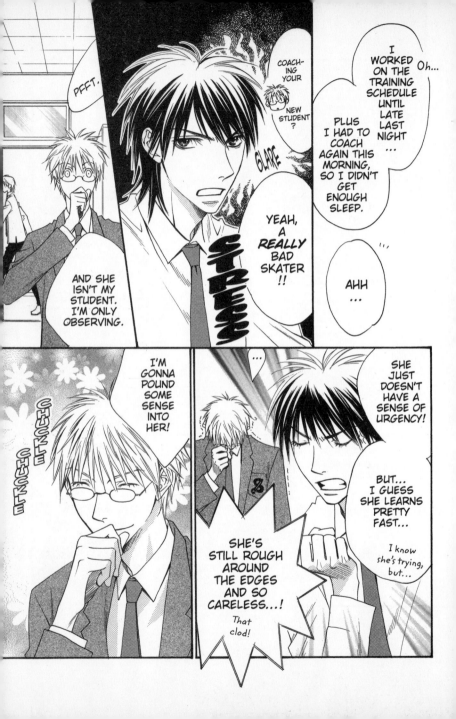

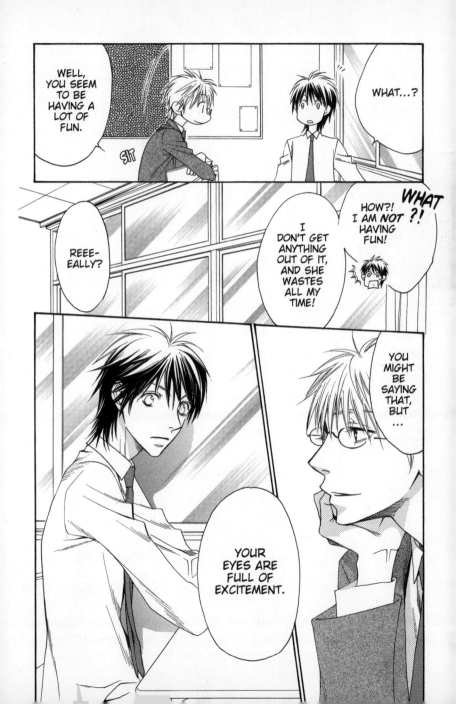

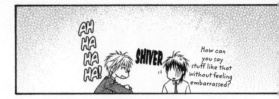

AH HA HA HA!

SHIVER

How can you say stuff like that without feeling embarrassed?

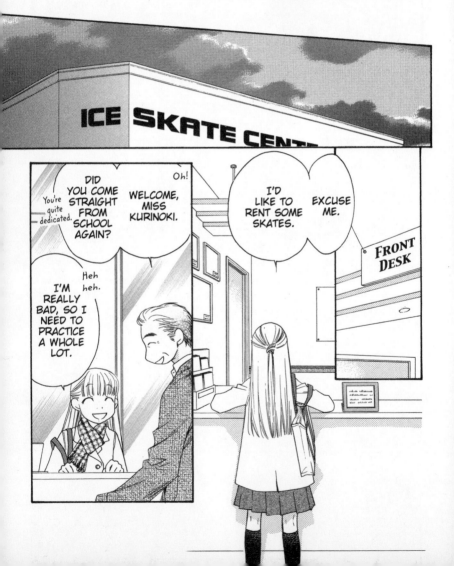

ICE SKATE CENTE

DID YOU COME STRAIGHT FROM SCHOOL AGAIN?

You're quite dedicated.

Oh! WELCOME, MISS KURINOKI.

I'D LIKE TO RENT SOME SKATES.

EXCUSE ME.

FRONT DESK

Heh heh.

I'M REALLY BAD, SO I NEED TO PRACTICE A WHOLE LOT.

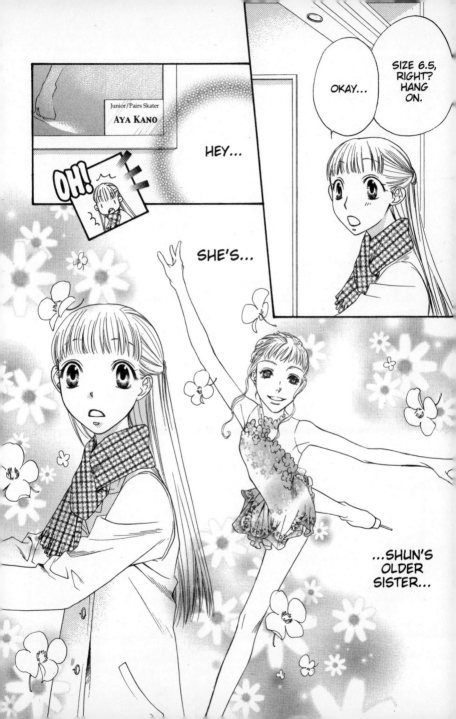

Junior/Pairs Skater
AYA KANO

OH!

SIZE 6.5,
RIGHT?
HANG
ON.

OKAY...

HEY...

SHE'S...

...SHUN'S
OLDER
SISTER...

SHE'S
...

MAAAA
...

...REALLY
PRETTY.

WHA—!

H
U
G

heh heh

...YAAAA!

DID I
SURPRISE
YOU?

Hee!

SHE
WAS A
REALLY
FANTASTIC
ATHLETE!

They
were
skating
partners.

SHE'S
SHUN'S
SISTER.

YOU
ALWAYS
COME
EARLY.

WHAT
WERE YOU
LOOKING
AT?

IT WAS
AWESOME
SEEING
THE TWO
OF THEM
SKATE AS
A PAIR.

HIKARU
...

THEY
FLOWED
TOGETHER
PERFECTLY
!

OH...

OH
...

YOU
MEAN OF
AYA?

Er...

I WAS
LOOKING
AT THE
PHOTOS
...

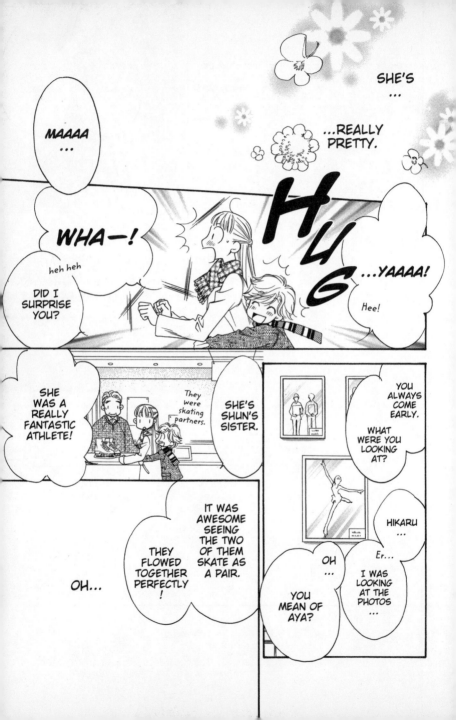

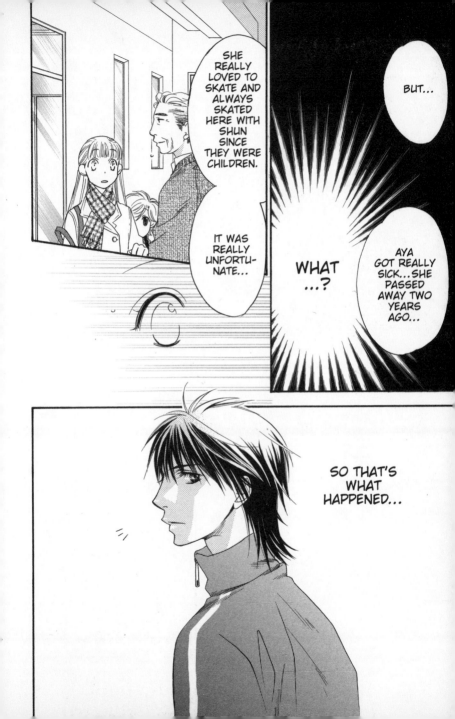

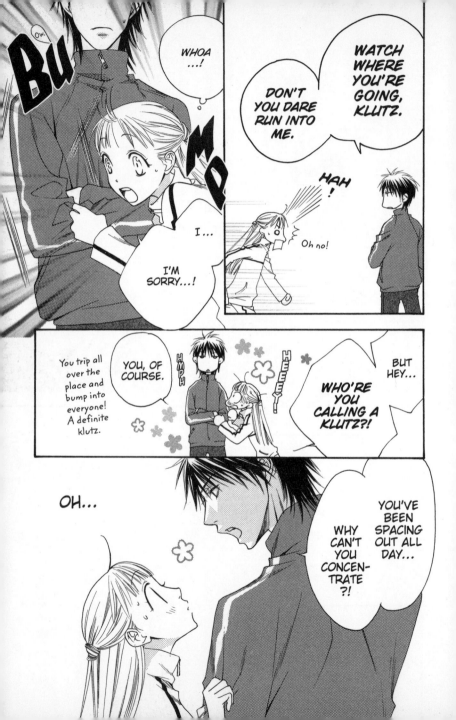

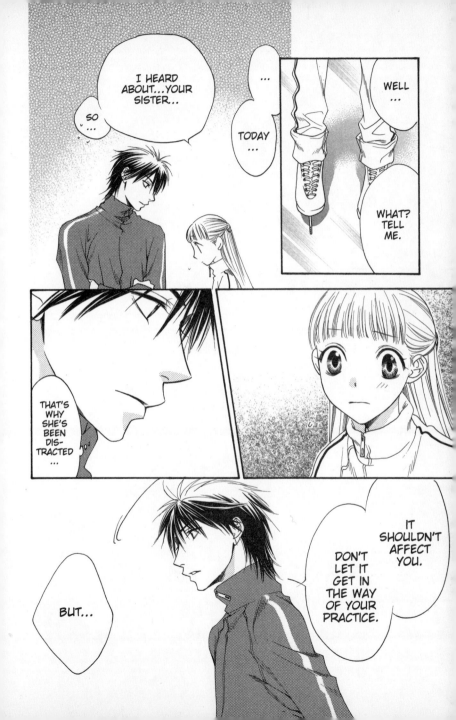

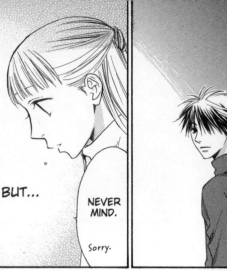

BMP

BUT...

NEVER
MIND.

Sorry.

BUT
THAT MUST
BE THE
REASON...

...HE ONLY
WANTS
TO DO
SINGLES...

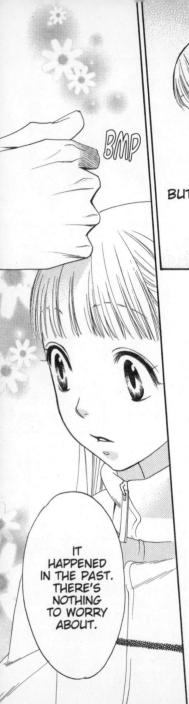

IT
HAPPENED
IN THE PAST.
THERE'S
NOTHING
TO WORRY
ABOUT.

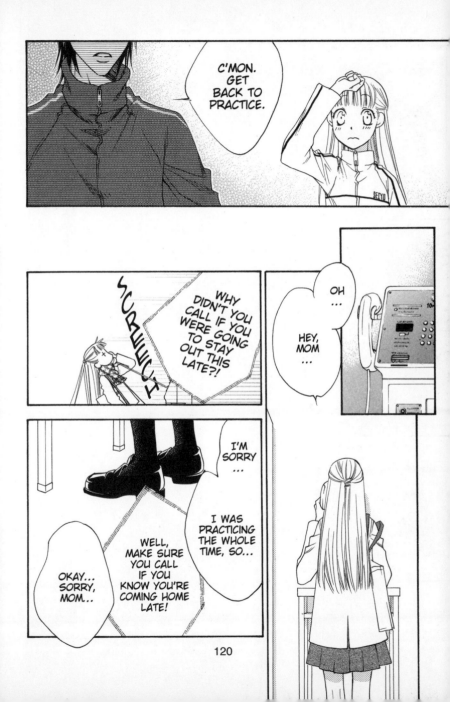

120

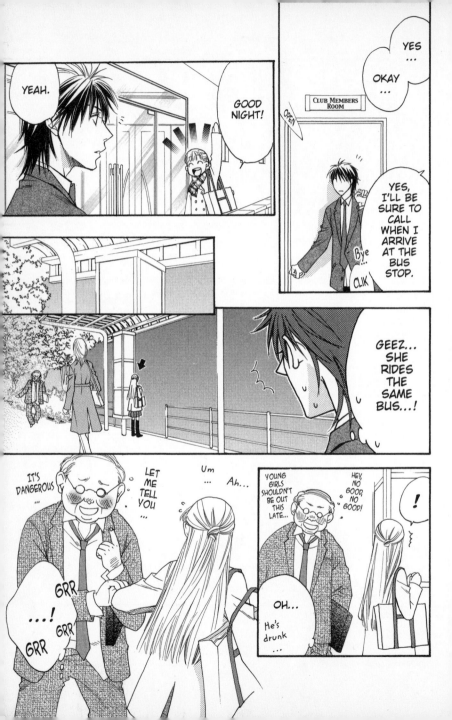

YEAH.

GOOD NIGHT!

YES
...

OKAY
...

CLUB MEMBERS ROOM

OPEN

YES, I'LL BE SURE TO CALL WHEN I ARRIVE AT THE BUS STOP.

Bye...

CLIK

GEEZ... SHE RIDES THE SAME BUS...!

IT'S DANGEROUS ...

LET ME TELL YOU ...

Um ... Ah...

YOUNG GIRLS SHOULDN'T BE OUT THIS LATE...

HEY, NO GOOD, NO GOOD!

!

OH...

He's drunk ...

...!

GRR

GRR

GRR

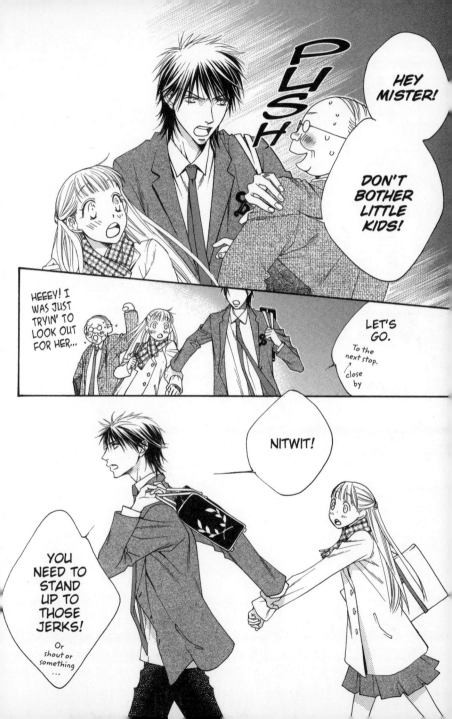

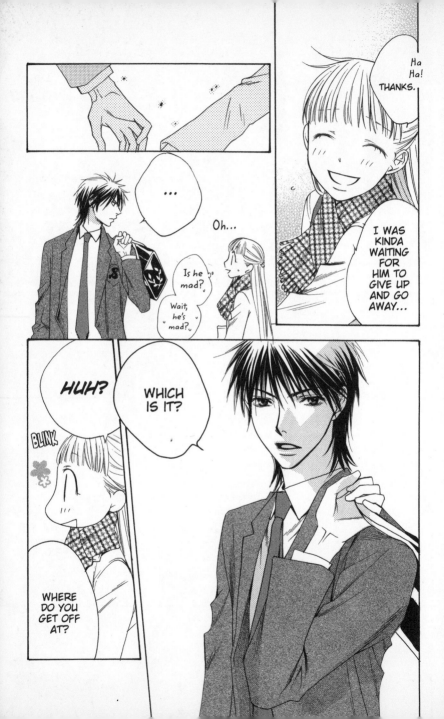

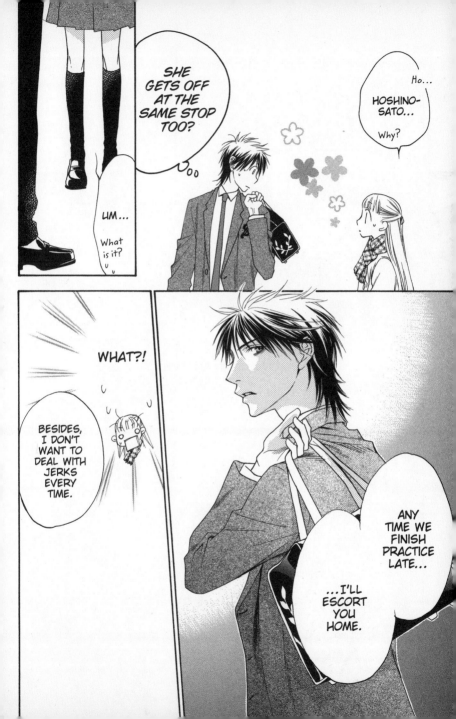

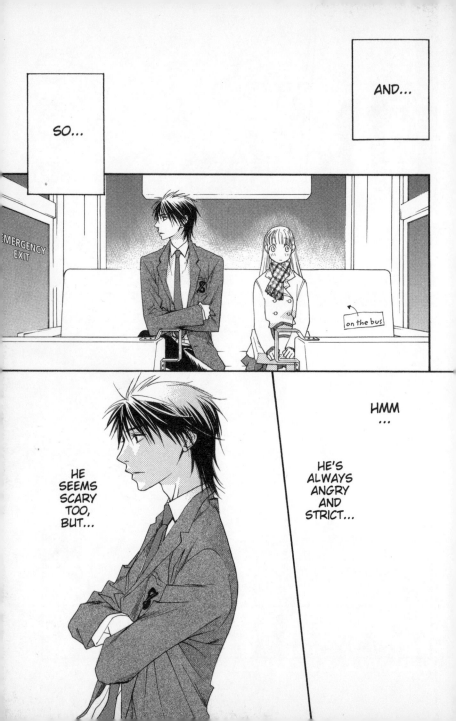

SO...

AND...

on the bus

HMM ...

HE'S ALWAYS ANGRY AND STRICT...

HE SEEMS SCARY TOO, BUT...

EMERGENCY EXIT

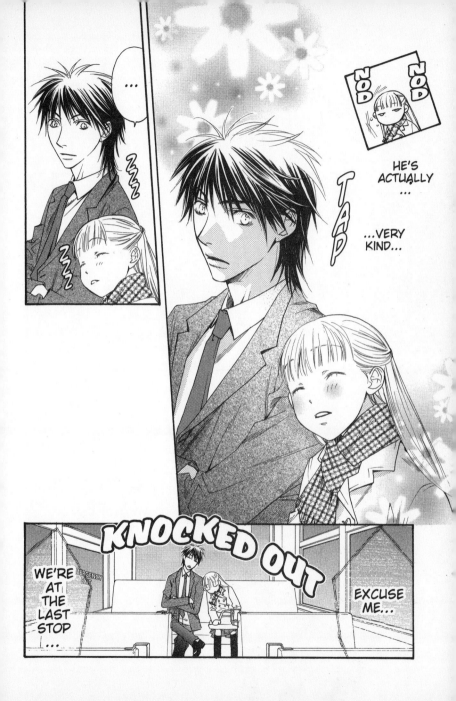

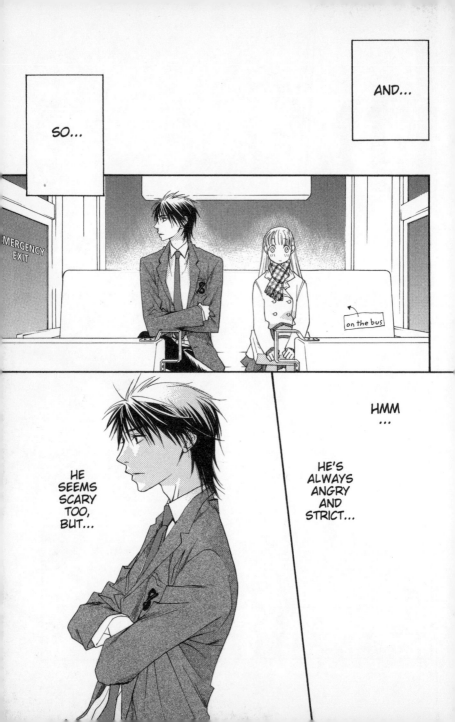

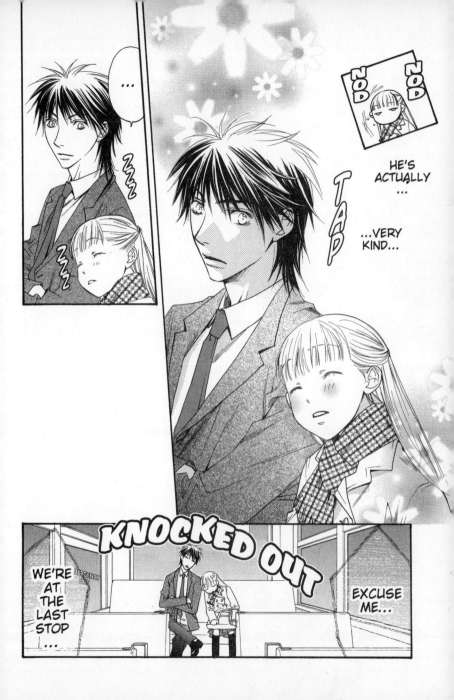

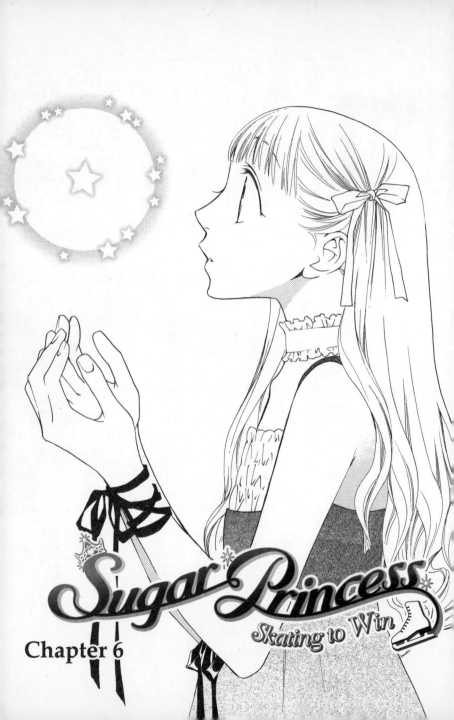

Sugar Princess
Skating to Win

Chapter 6

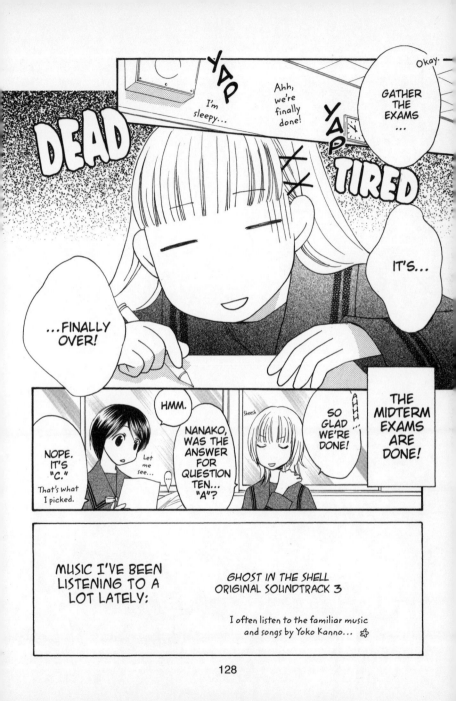

MUSIC I'VE BEEN
LISTENING TO A
LOT LATELY:

GHOST IN THE SHELL
ORIGINAL SOUNDTRACK 3

I often listen to the familiar music
and songs by Yoko Kanno...

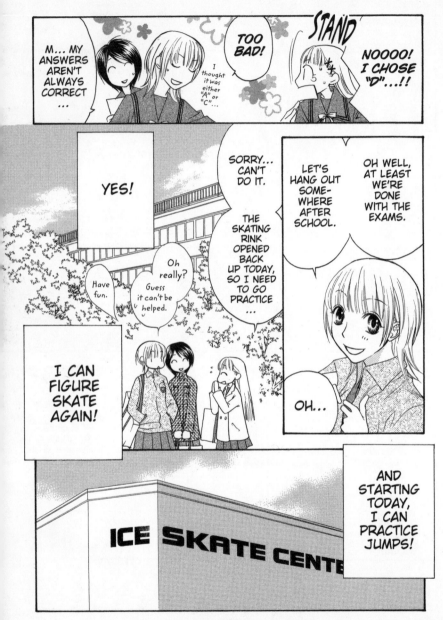

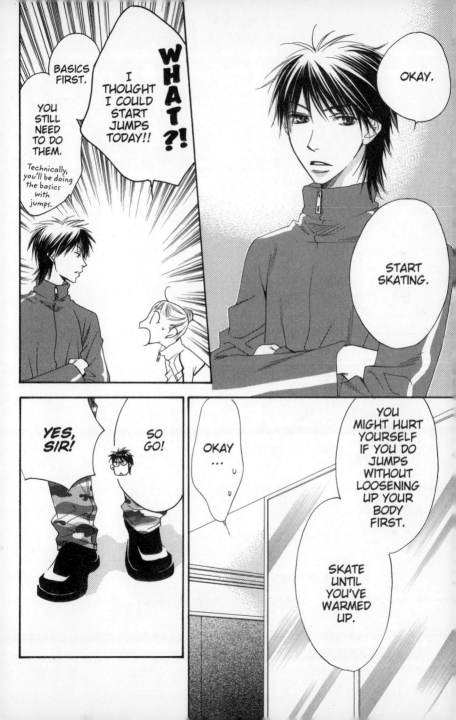

BASICS FIRST.

I THOUGHT I COULD START JUMPS TODAY!!

WHAT?!

OKAY.

YOU STILL NEED TO DO THEM.

Technically, you'll be doing the basics with jumps.

START SKATING.

YES, SIR!

SO GO!

OKAY...

YOU MIGHT HURT YOURSELF IF YOU DO JUMPS WITHOUT LOOSENING UP YOUR BODY FIRST.

SKATE UNTIL YOU'VE WARMED UP.

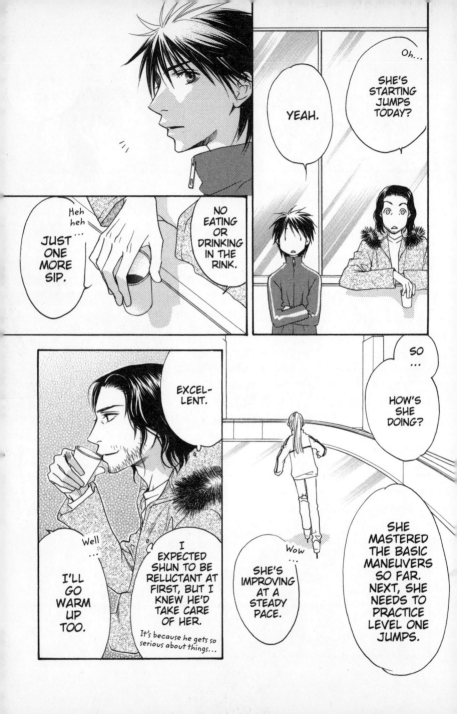

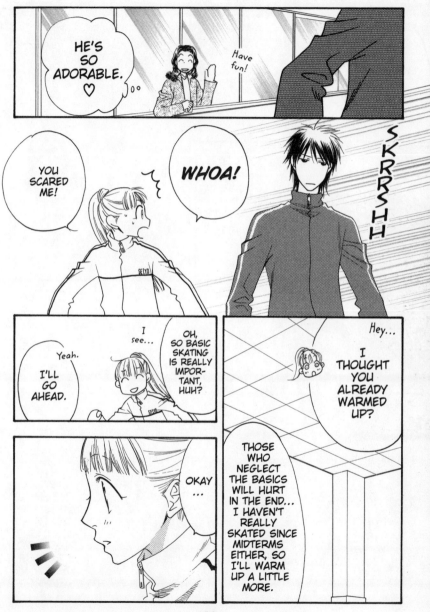

132

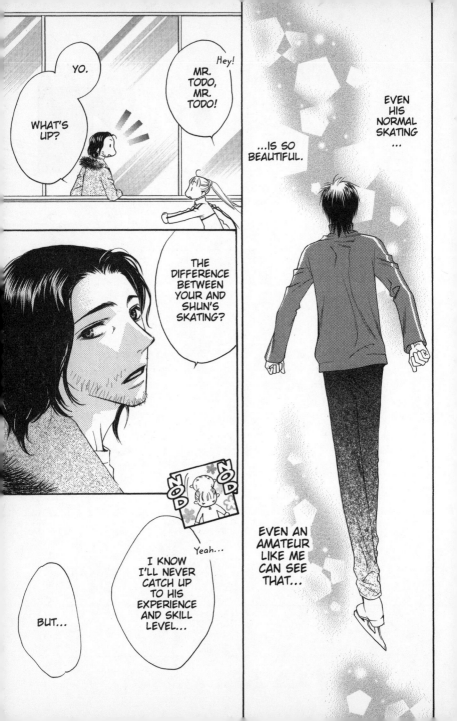

YO.

Hey!

MR. TODO, MR. TODO!

WHAT'S UP?

THE DIFFERENCE BETWEEN YOUR AND SHUN'S SKATING?

NOD NOD

Yeah...

I KNOW I'LL NEVER CATCH UP TO HIS EXPERIENCE AND SKILL LEVEL...

BUT...

EVEN HIS NORMAL SKATING ...

...IS SO BEAUTIFUL.

EVEN AN AMATEUR LIKE ME CAN SEE THAT...

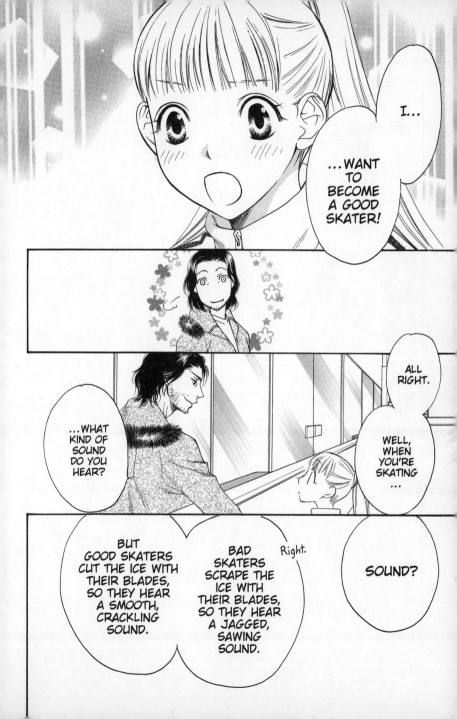

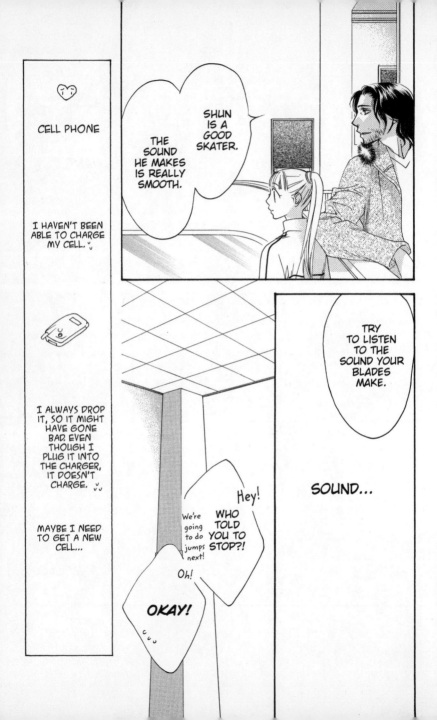

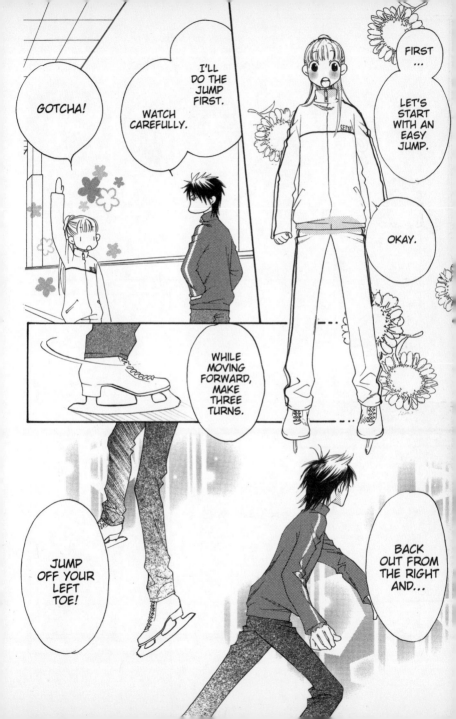

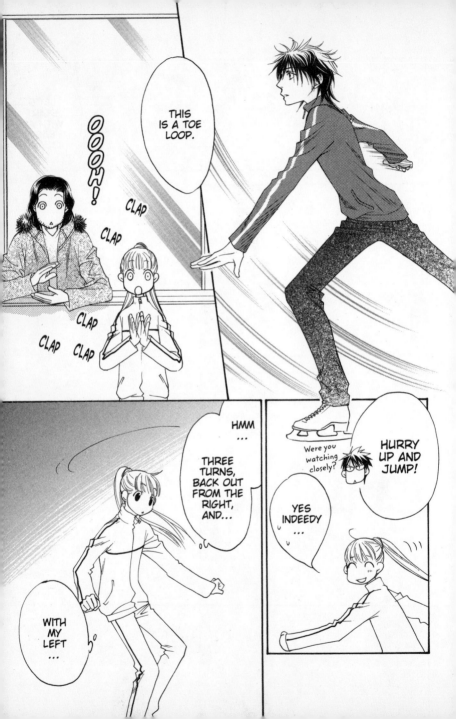

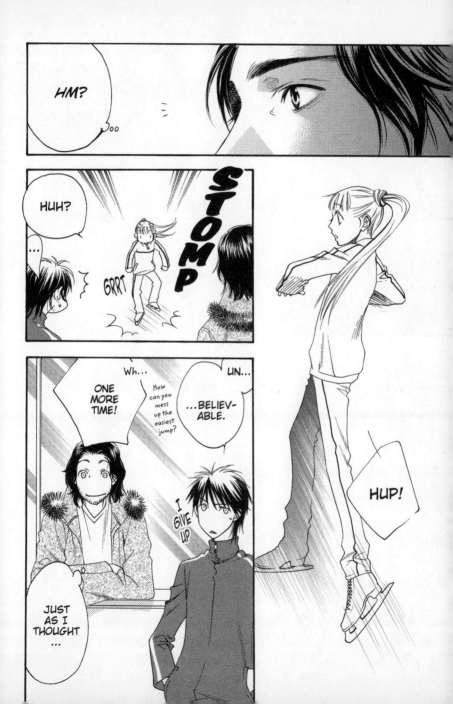

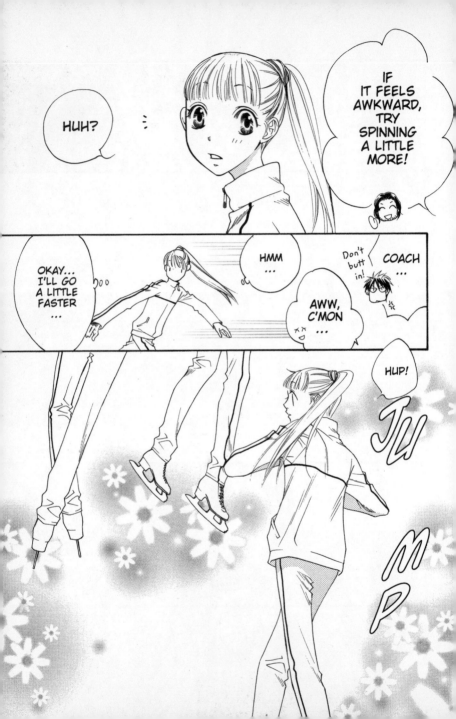

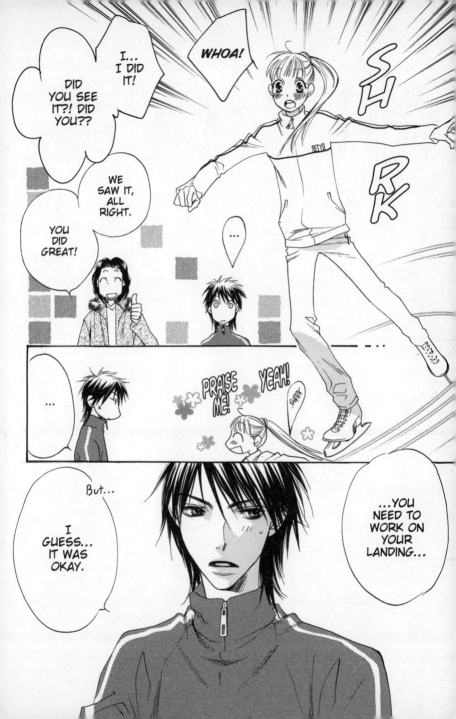

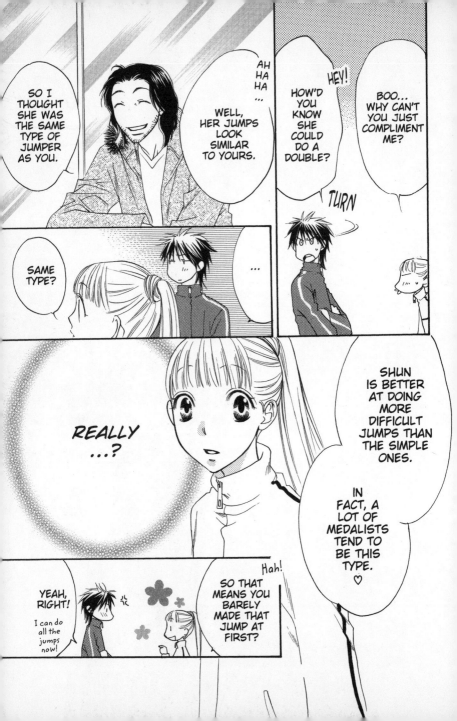

Men's Singles

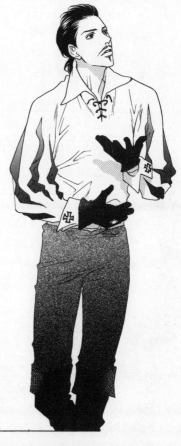

He's very entertaining! I like how he entertains his audience! The illustration to the right is when he performed as d'Artagnan of the Three Musketeers. ☆

Philippe CANDELORO

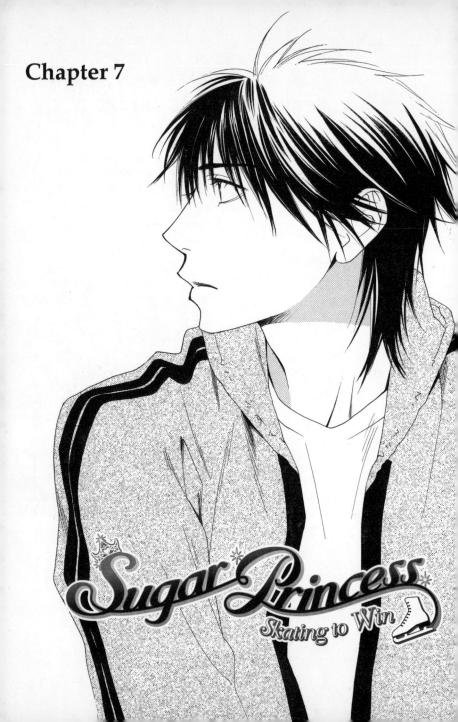

Chapter 7

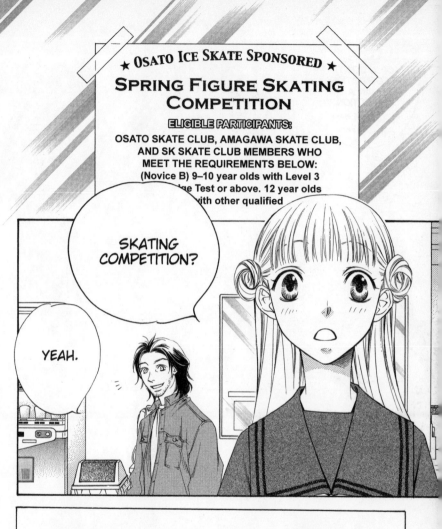

★ OSATO ICE SKATE SPONSORED ★

SPRING FIGURE SKATING COMPETITION

ELIGIBLE PARTICIPANTS:
OSATO SKATE CLUB, AMAGAWA SKATE CLUB, AND SK SKATE CLUB MEMBERS WHO MEET THE REQUIREMENTS BELOW: (Novice B) 9–10 year olds with Level 3 ___ge Test or above. 12 year olds ___ith other qualified

SKATING COMPETITION?

YEAH.

A SCARY INCIDENT THAT HAPPENED RECENTLY

WHEN I SAW THIS BROWN, CRAWLY THING (COCKROACH) HANGING OUT OF THE MOUTH OF MY CAT (SUE)... SHIVER

Where did she even find it?!

HMPH.

PROUD

To make things worse, it was like she brought the horrible thing to me to show it off...

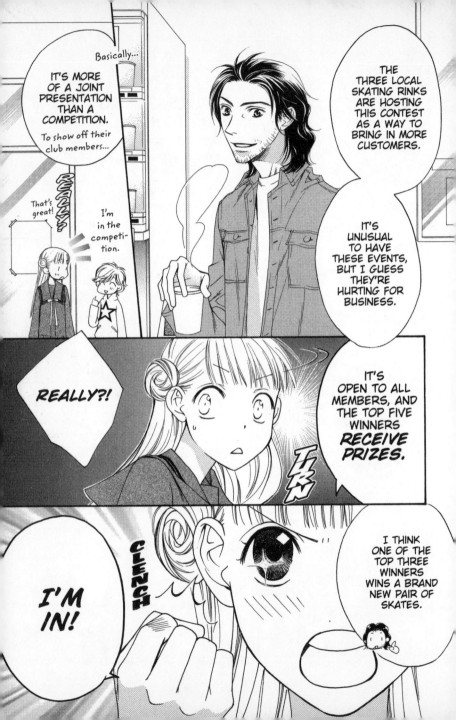

THE THREE LOCAL SKATING RINKS ARE HOSTING THIS CONTEST AS A WAY TO BRING IN MORE CUSTOMERS.

Basically...

IT'S MORE OF A JOINT PRESENTATION THAN A COMPETITION.

To show off their club members...

IT'S UNUSUAL TO HAVE THESE EVENTS, BUT I GUESS THEY'RE HURTING FOR BUSINESS.

That's great!

I'm in the competi-tion.

REALLY?!

IT'S OPEN TO ALL MEMBERS, AND THE TOP FIVE WINNERS *RECEIVE PRIZES.*

TUKN

I'M IN!

CLENCH

I THINK ONE OF THE TOP THREE WINNERS WINS A BRAND NEW PAIR OF SKATES.

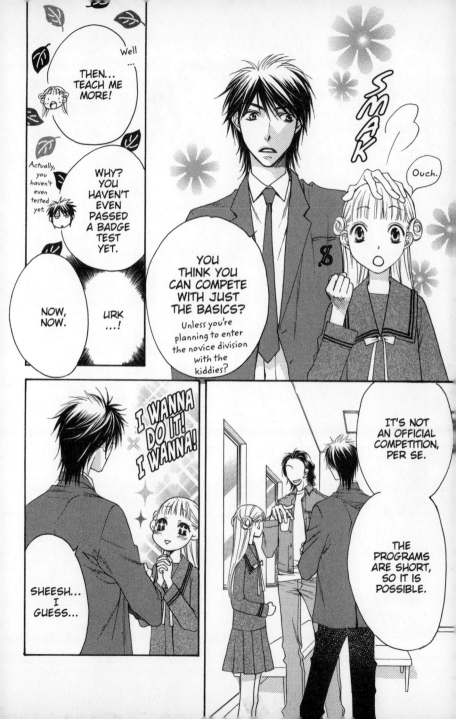

Well...

THEN... TEACH ME MORE!

WHY? YOU HAVEN'T EVEN PASSED A BADGE TEST YET.

Actually, you haven't even tested yet.

NOW, NOW.

URK...!

YOU THINK YOU CAN COMPETE WITH JUST THE BASICS? Unless you're planning to enter the novice division with the kiddies?

SMAK

Ouch.

I WANNA DO IT! I WANNA!

SHEESH... I GUESS...

IT'S NOT AN OFFICIAL COMPETITION, PER SE.

THE PROGRAMS ARE SHORT, SO IT IS POSSIBLE.

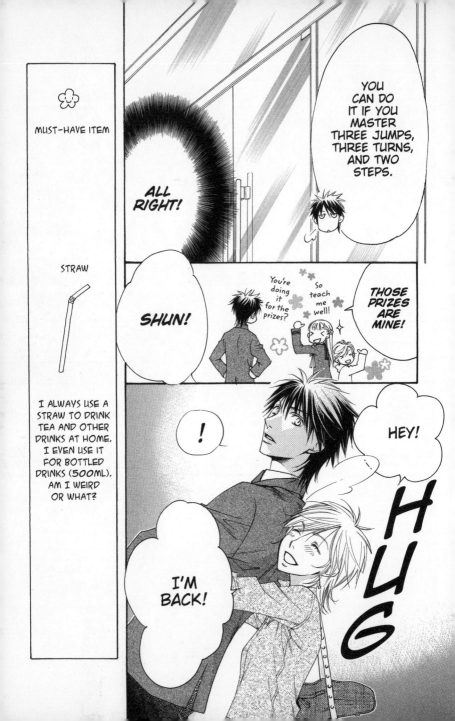

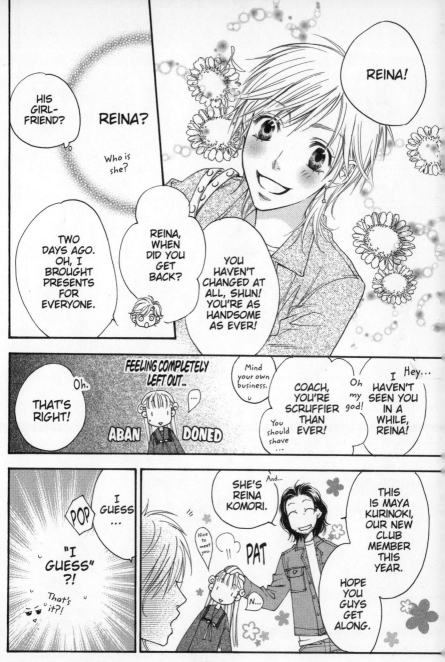

HIS GIRL-FRIEND?

REINA?

Who is she?

REINA!

TWO DAYS AGO. OH, I BROUGHT PRESENTS FOR EVERYONE.

REINA, WHEN DID YOU GET BACK?

YOU HAVEN'T CHANGED AT ALL, SHUN! YOU'RE AS HANDSOME AS EVER!

Oh.

FEELING COMPLETELY LEFT OUT...

THAT'S RIGHT!

...

ABAN DONED

Mind your own business.

COACH, YOU'RE SCRUFFIER THAN EVER!

You should shave...

Oh my god!

I HAVEN'T SEEN YOU IN A WHILE, REINA!

Hey...

POP

I GUESS...

"I GUESS"?!

That's it?!

SHE'S REINA KOMORI.

And...

Nice to meet you.

PAT

N...

THIS IS MAYA KURINOKI, OUR NEW CLUB MEMBER THIS YEAR.

HOPE YOU GUYS GET ALONG.

148

AS A And! REWARD FOR GETTING INTO A GOOD HIGH SCHOOL, HER FATHER TOOK HER AND THE REST OF THE FAMILY TO GUAM.

SO SHE'S ALSO A CLUB MEMBER...

IT WASN'T TOO HOT. I BROUGHT PRESENTS!

WELCOME BACK! HOW WAS GUAM?!

YAY!

HEY.

REINA!

YAY!

YAP

YAP

YA P

Good afternoon!

OH...

So...

HER WHOLE FAMILY WENT OVERSEAS... I'M JEALOUS!

Ugh.

My family could never afford that.

You know...

REINA'S A CLUB MEMBER TOO.

POKE POKE

She doesn't know me, after all...

Sigh

OH WELL...

Wooow!

REINA, THAT'S SO BEAUTIFUL!

I CAN'T BELIEVE YOU HAVEN'T SKATED IN MONTHS!

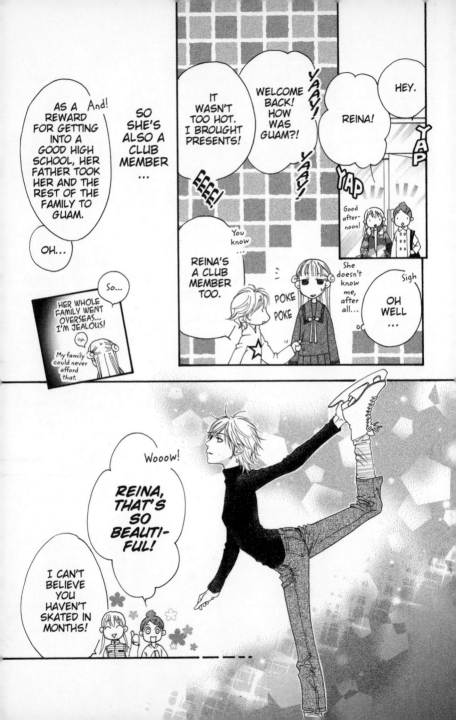

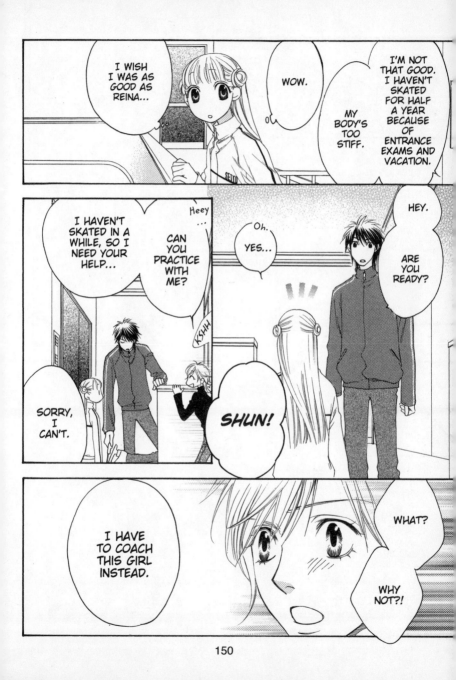

150

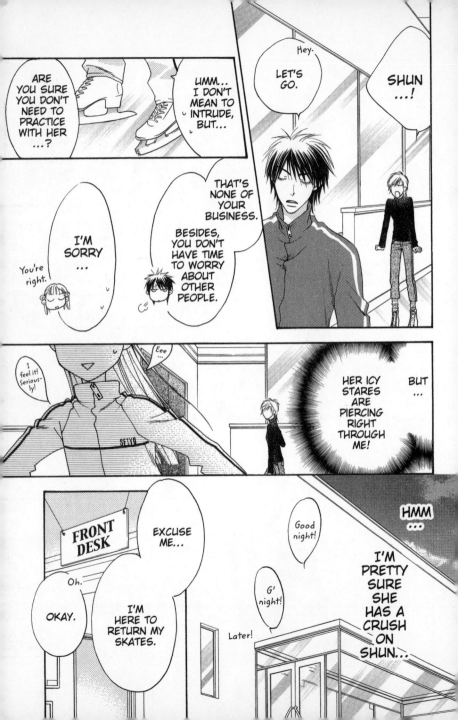

ARE YOU SURE YOU DON'T NEED TO PRACTICE WITH HER ...?

UMM... I DON'T MEAN TO INTRUDE, BUT...

Hey.

LET'S GO.

SHUN ...!

THAT'S NONE OF YOUR BUSINESS.

BESIDES, YOU DON'T HAVE TIME TO WORRY ABOUT OTHER PEOPLE.

I'M SORRY ...

You're right.

I feel it! Seriously!

Eee ...

HER ICY STARES ARE PIERCING RIGHT THROUGH ME!

BUT ...

FRONT DESK

EXCUSE ME...

Oh.

OKAY.

I'M HERE TO RETURN MY SKATES.

Good night!

G' night!

Later!

HMM ...

I'M PRETTY SURE SHE HAS A CRUSH ON SHUN...

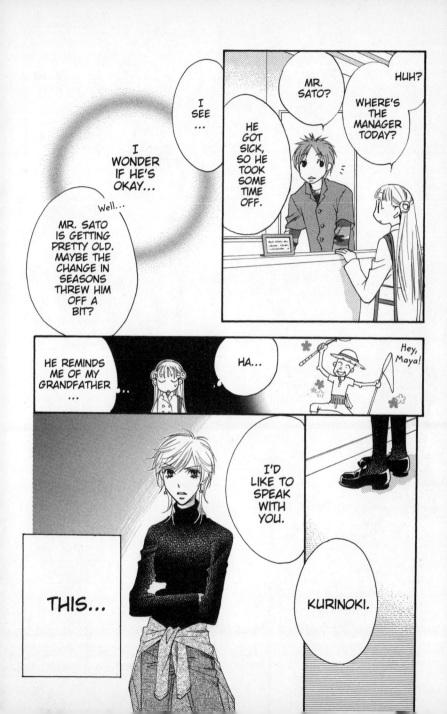

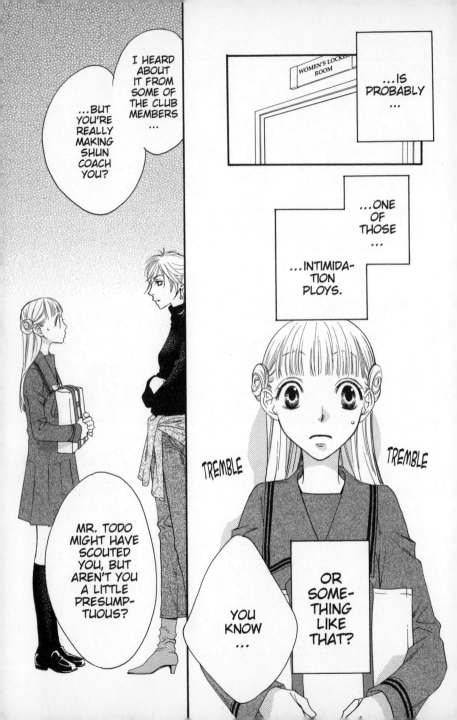

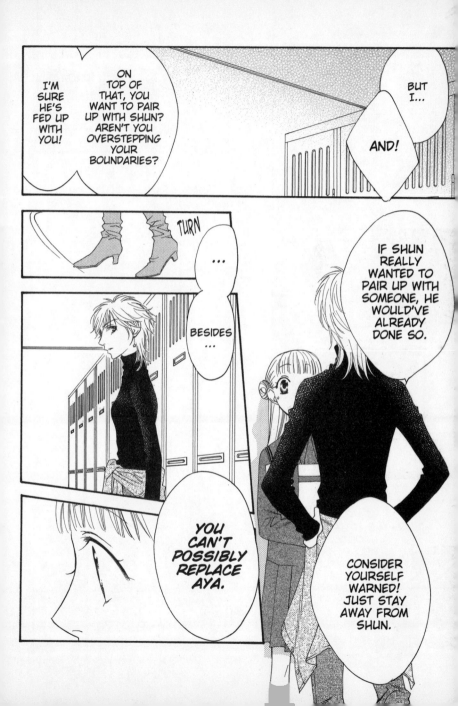

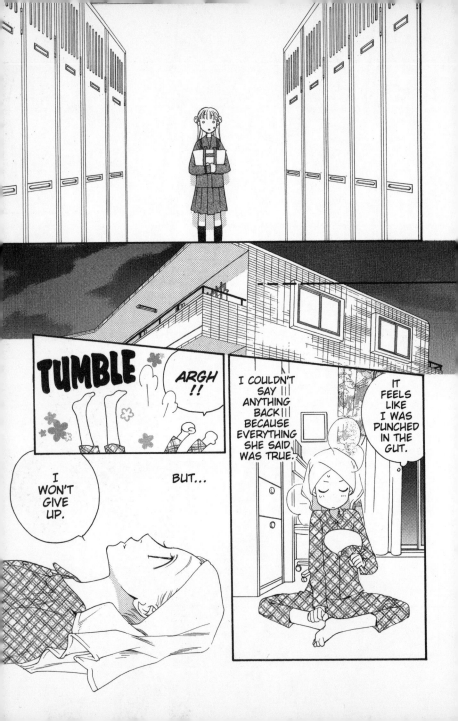

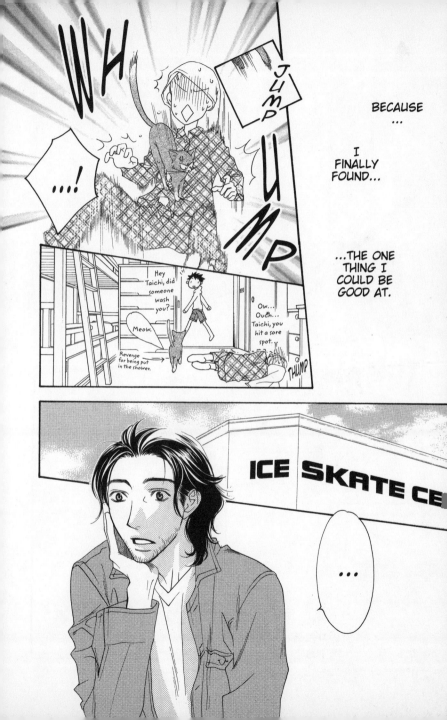

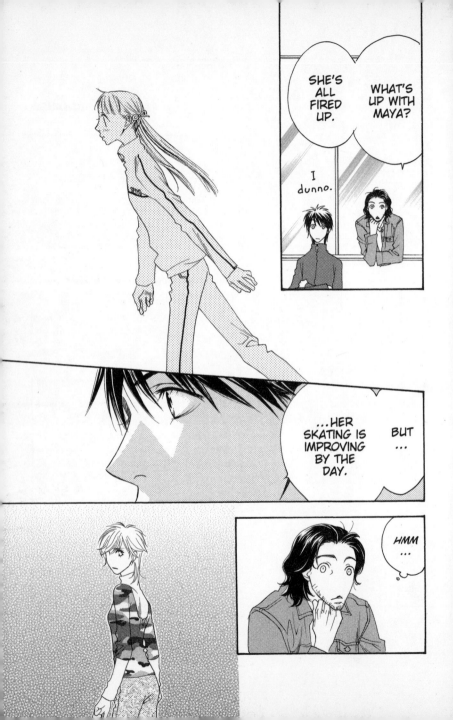

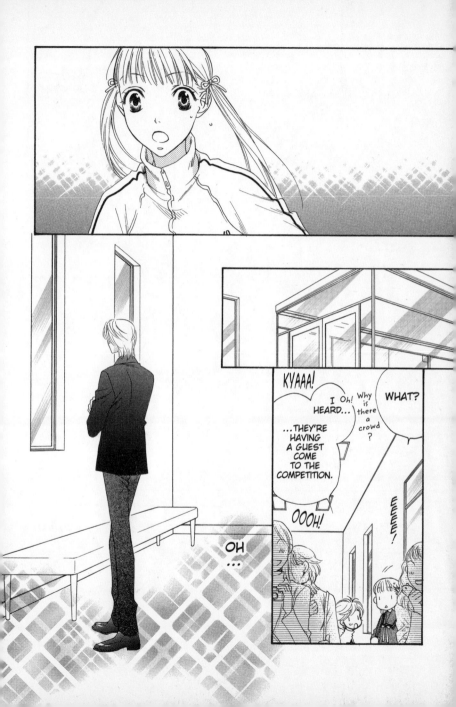

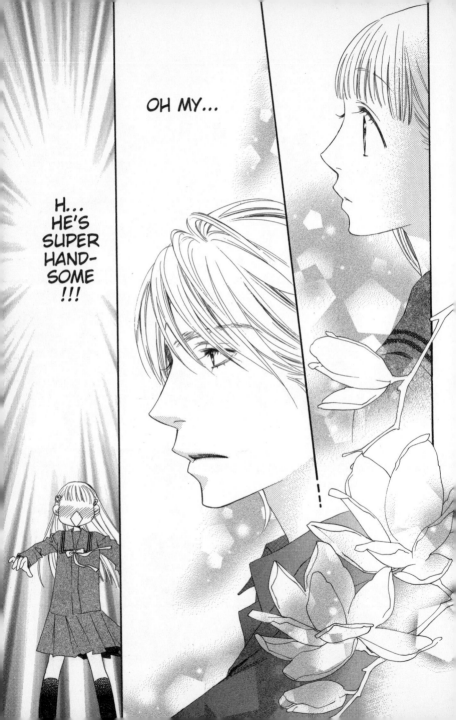

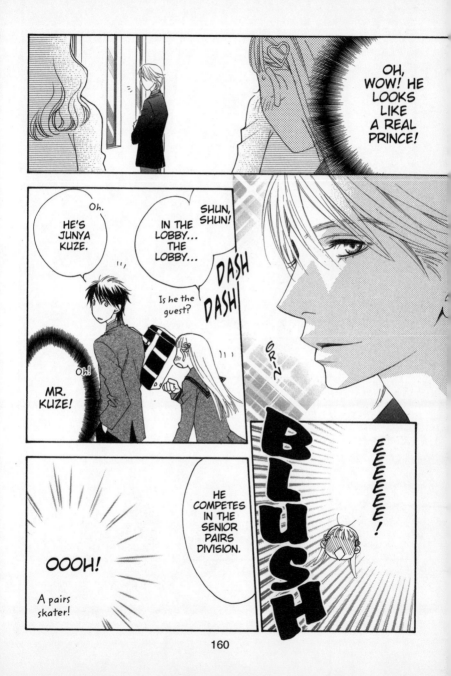

Chapter 8

OH, WOW! HE LOOKS LIKE A REAL PRINCE!

HE'S JUNYA KUZE.

Oh.

SHUN, SHUN! IN THE LOBBY... THE LOBBY...

Is he the guest?

DASH DASH!

OH!

MR. KUZE!

GRIN

BLUSH

EEEEEE!

HE COMPETES IN THE SENIOR PAIRS DIVISION.

OOOH!

A pairs skater!

160

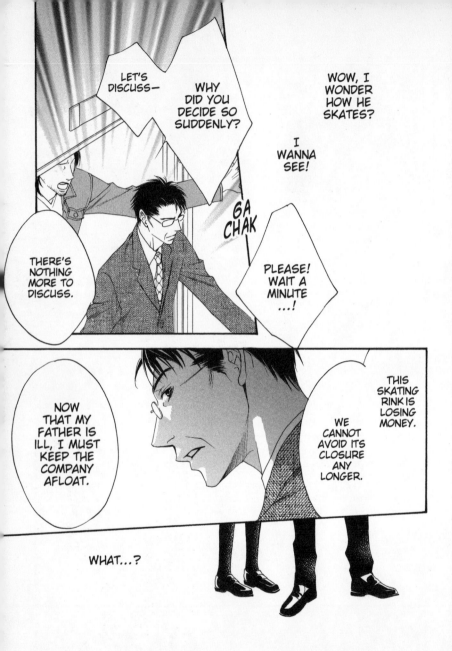

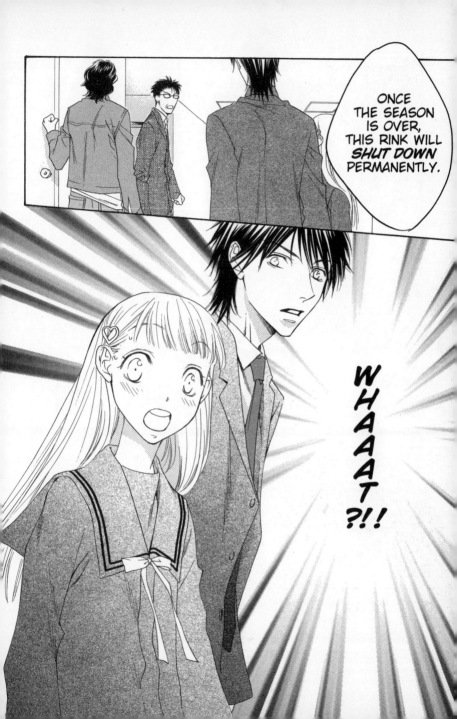

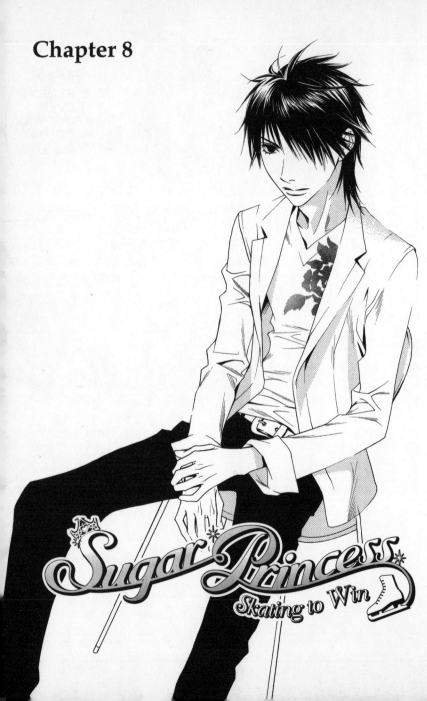

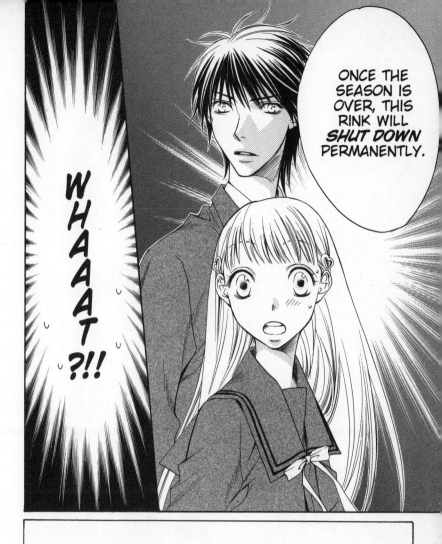

MUSIC THAT I'M
LISTENING TO LATELY:

MIKA NAKASHIMA.

I've listened to her since her debut!
Not only do I love the way she
looks, but her voice is amazing too!

I heard somewhere that she owns the same type of cat as me (Somalian), so I somehow feel close to her!

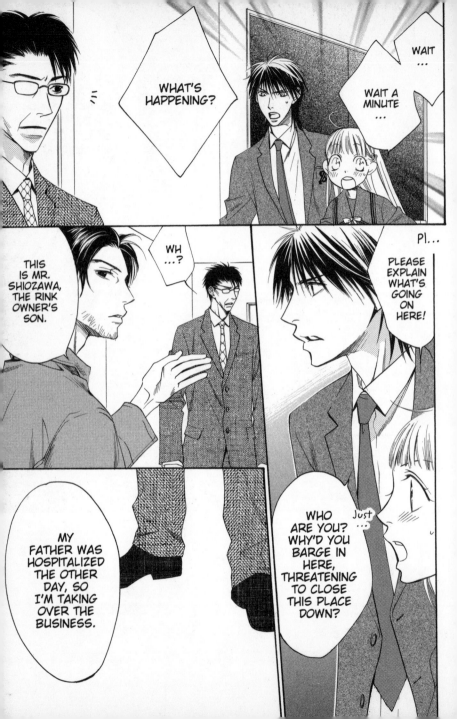

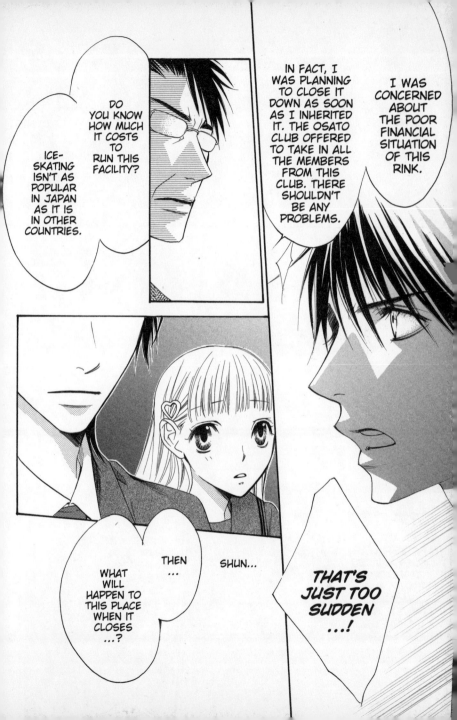

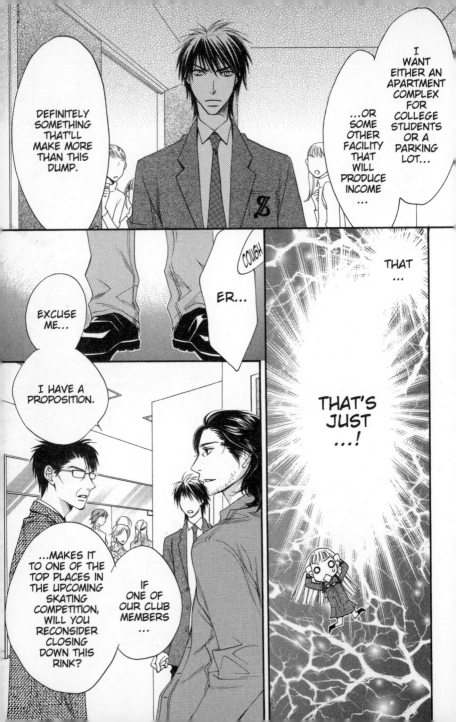

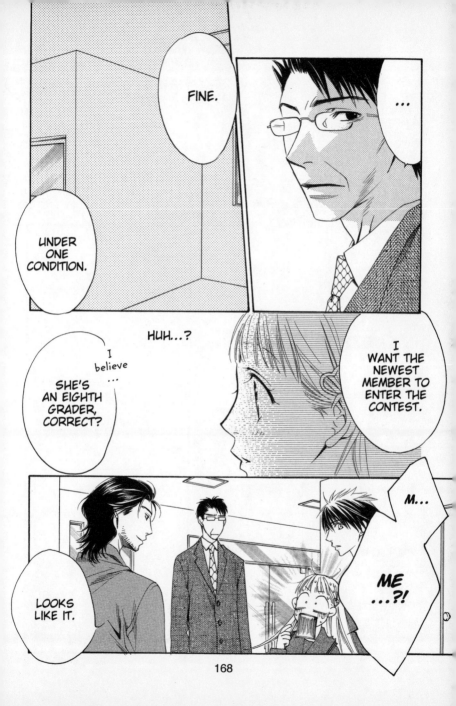

168

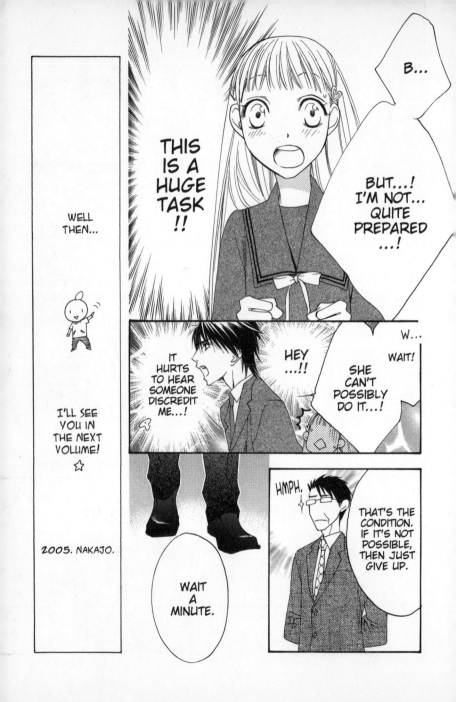

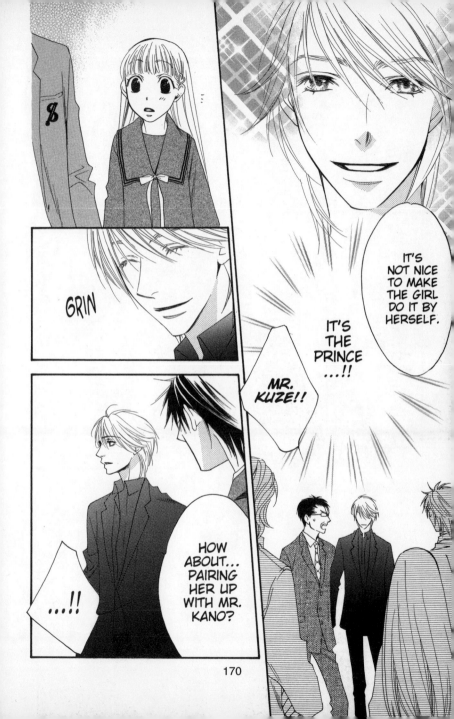

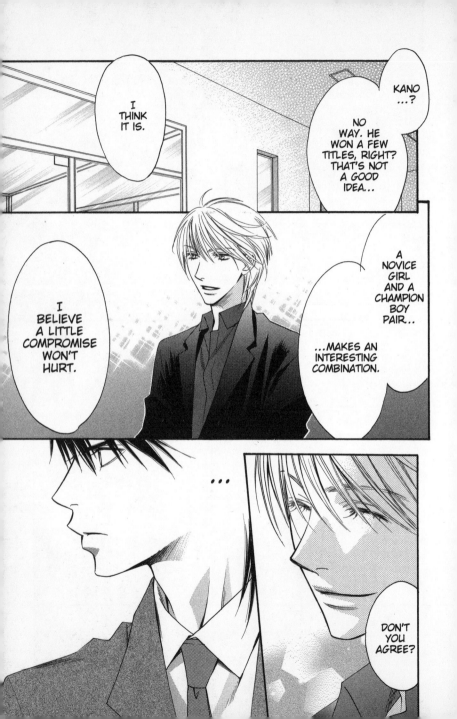

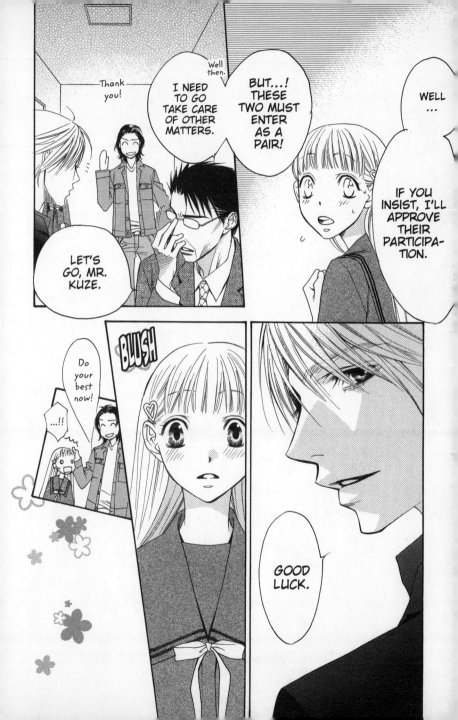

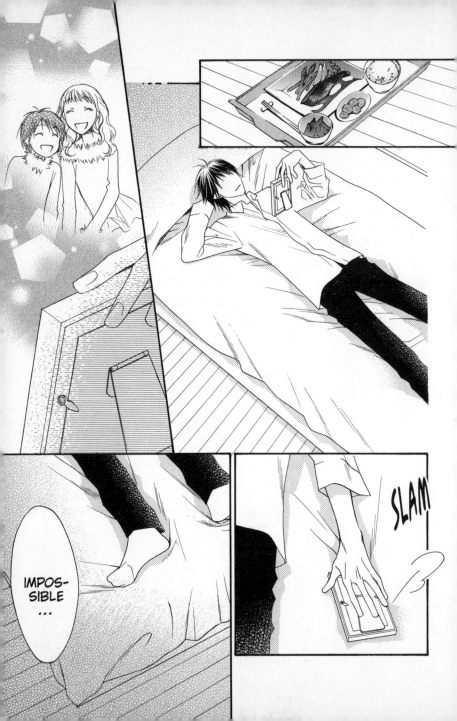

IMPOS-
SIBLE
...

SLAM

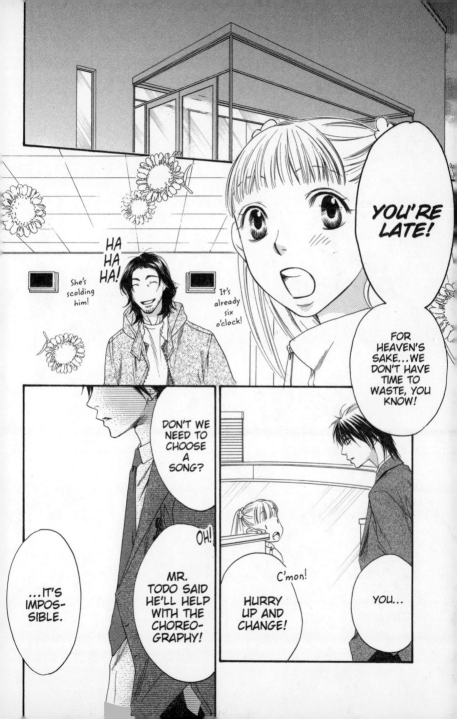

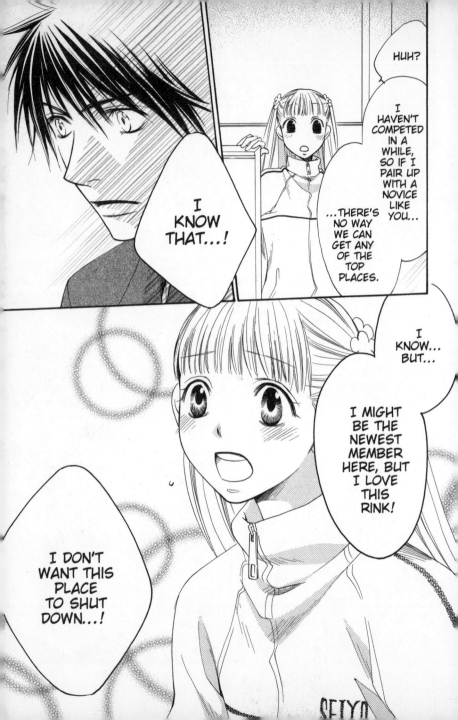

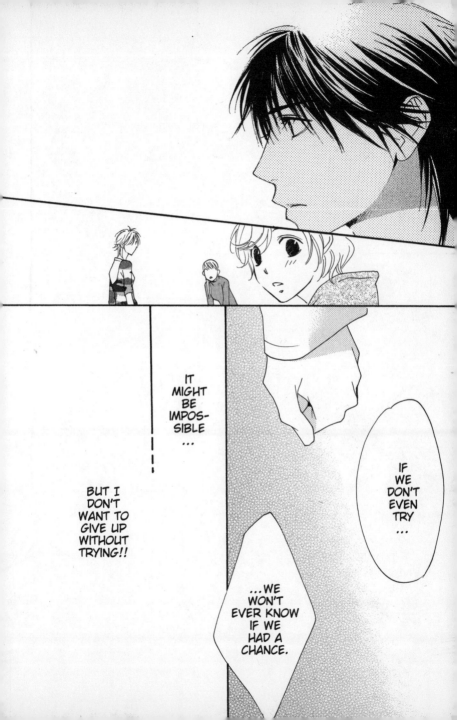

IT MIGHT BE IMPOSSIBLE...

IF WE DON'T EVEN TRY...

BUT I DON'T WANT TO GIVE UP WITHOUT TRYING!!

...WE WON'T EVER KNOW IF WE HAD A CHANCE.

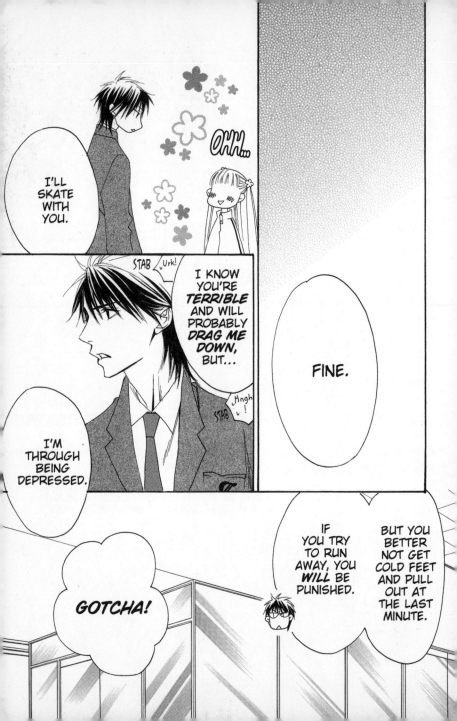

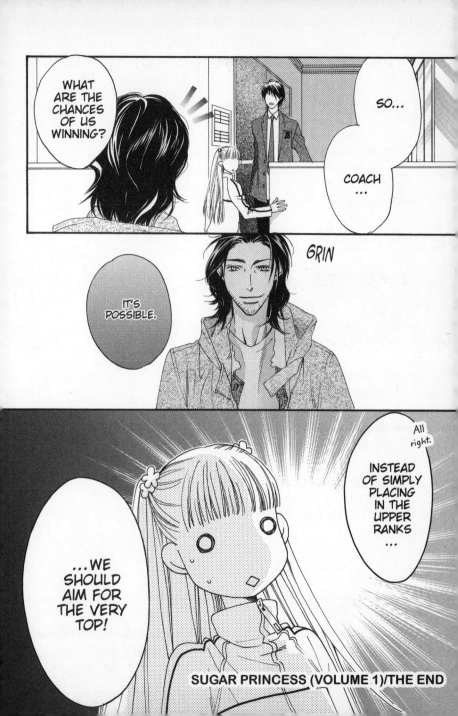

SUGAR PRINCESS (VOLUME 1)/THE END

THANK YOU FOR ALL YOUR HELP!

INTERVIEWS:

★ Jin Sano (Meiji Temple Ice Skate Center Instructor)

★ Takako Saito (ice blue)

★ And all the other coaches and athletes!

REFERENCE MATERIAL:

★ *Figure Skating Magic* by Kyoko Umeda and Tomoko Imagawa (Bungei Shunbun)

★ *Fumio Igarashi's Graceful Figure Skating* by Kazumi Shiraishi (Shinshokan)

★ "World Figure Skating" in *Dance Magazine* (Shinshokan)

★ "Invitation to Figure Skating" in *Dance Magazine* (Shinshokan)

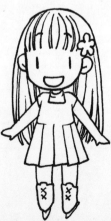

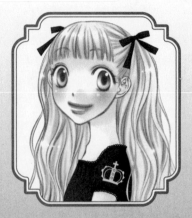

Hisaya Nakajo's manga series *Hanazakari no Kimitachi he* (For You in Full Blossom, casually known as *Hana-Kimi*) has been a hit since it first appeared in 1997 in the shojo manga magazine *Hana to Yume* (Flowers and Dreams). In Japan, a *Hana-Kimi* art book and several drama CDs have been released. Her other manga series include *Missing Piece* (two volumes) and *Yumemiru Happa* (The Dreaming Leaf, one volume).

Sugar Princess
Vol. 1
The Shojo Beat Manga Edition

This manga volume contains material that was originally published in English in *Shojo Beat* magazine, July 2008 issue. Artwork in the magazine may have been altered slightly from what is presented in this volume.

STORY & ART BY
HISAYA NAKAJO

Translation & Adaptation/Anastasia Moreno
Touch-up Art & Lettering/Rina Mapa
Design/Izumi Hirayama
Editor/Amy Yu

Editor in Chief, Books/Alvin Lu
Editor in Chief, Magazines/Marc Weidenbaum
VP of Publishing Licensing/Rika Inouye
VP of Sales/Gonzalo Ferreyra
Sr. VP of Marketing/Liza Coppola
Publisher/Hyoe Narita

Sugar Princess by Hisaya Nakajo
© Hisaya Nakajo 2005
All rights reserved.
First published in Japan in 2005 by HAKUSENSHA, Inc., Tokyo.
English language translation rights arranged with Hakusensha, Inc., Tokyo
The stories, characters and incidents mentioned in this publication are
entirely fictional.

Printed in Canada

Published by VIZ Media, LLC
P.O. Box 77010
San Francisco, CA 94107

Shojo Beat Manga Edition
10 9 8 7 6 5 4 3 2 1
First printing, August 2008

www.viz.com

store.viz.com

PARENTAL ADVISORY
SUGAR PRINCESS is
rated A and is suitable
for readers of all ages.
ratings.viz.com

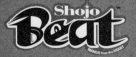

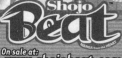
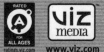

SB Tell us what you think about Shojo Beat Manga!

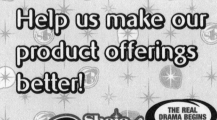